FRCS
General Surgery Section 1
Practice Questions

Roland Fernandes

FRCS MBBS BSc

First published in 2019 by Libri Publishing

ISBN 978-1-911450-44-3

A CIP catalogue record for this book is available from The British Library

Cover and Design by Carnegie Publishing

Printed in the UK by Severn

Libri Publishing
Brunel House
Volunteer Way
Faringdon
Oxfordshire
SN7 7YR

Tel: +44 (0)845 873 3837

www.libripublishing.co.uk

CONTENTS

CHAPTER 1
LESIONS OF THE SKIN AND SUBCUTANEOUS TISSUE

Answers on page 199–202

Dr Jonathan Slater

MBBS BSc MRCGP SCE Derm
Associate Specialist Dermatology
Surrey & Sussex Healthcare NHS Trust

Question 1

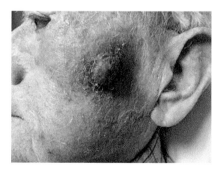

An elderly patient presents with this rapidly growing tender lesion on his left cheek.

a) Which of the following is the **least** likely diagnosis?

- A) Amelanotic melanoma
- B) Squamous cell carcinoma
- C) Merkel cell carcinoma
- D) Cutaneous metastasis
- E) Infected epidermoid cyst

b) What treatment option should you recommend?

    A) Radiotherapy

    B) Curettage and cautery

    C) Shave excision

    D) Excision with a 4mm margin

    E) Excision with a 6mm margin

Question 2

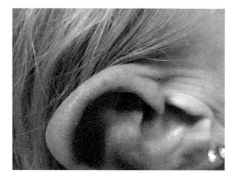

This lady presents to you with a painful lesion on the left ear proximal helix. Which element of her history is the most important in this case?

    A) Smoking history

    B) Past history of skin cancer

    C) Left hip and shoulder pains

    D) History of excess sun exposure

    E) History of weight loss

Question 3

Which layer of the skin is often described as a brick-and-mortar model with protein-rich cells surrounded by an extracellular lipid-rich matrix providing mechanical protection and impermeability?

    A) Stratum corneum

    B) Stratum basale

    C) Stratum granulosum

    D) Stratum lucidum

    E) Stratum spinosum

Question 4

Which of the following is not a pre-malignant lesion?

    A) Extramammary Paget's disease

    B) Bowen's disease

    C) Cutaneous horn

    D) Adenoma sebaceum

    E) Giant congenital pigmented naevus

Question 5

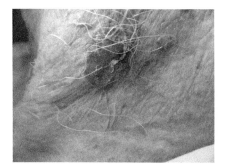

On reviewing a surgical patient you notice the lesion shown in the image above on the patient's neck. Which of the following is not a recommended treatment option?

    A) Primary surgical excision and closure

    B) Excision and closure with a local flap

    C) Radiotherapy

    D) Treatment with a Hedgehog inhibitor

    E) Excision and full thickness skin grafting

Question 6

Which of the following is false with regard to basal cell carcinomas of the skin?

    A) UV radiation is a strong risk factor

    B) Mainly affects Caucasian people

    C) Incidence is highest near equator

    D) Usually slow growing

    E) More common in women

Question 7

Which of the following are examples of high-risk BCCs?

A) Lesions with ill-defined margins

B) Lesions on the nose

C) Recurrent lesions

D) Lesions greater than 20mm

E) All the above

Question 8

Which of the following is the least acceptable treatment for superficial BCCs in an otherwise-healthy young patient?

A) 5 Fluoruracil (Efudix)

B) Moh's micrographic surgery

C) Radiotherapy

D) Photodynamic therapy

E) Surgical excision

Question 9

A patient with a metallic heart valve is on your surgical list for excision of a basal cell carcinoma. Which antibiotic prophylaxis do you commence?

A) Single-dose penicillin an hour prior to the procedure

B) A week's course of penicillin after the procedure

C) Delay until you have discussed his case with a cardiologist

D) No antibiotic propylaxis

E) A week's course of erythromycin

Question 10

Which of the following is used to determine prognosis in squamous cell cancer (SCC)?

A) Blumgart grade

B) Breslow thickness

C) Broder's grade

D) Bloom–Richardson grade

E) Fuhrman grade

Question 11

What is the minimum clinical excision margin for a well-defined, low-risk 16mm SCC?

    A) 2mm

    B) 4mm

    C) 6mm

    D) 8mm

    E) 10mm

Question 12

What is the minimum excision margin for a primary clinically well-defined low-risk BCC?

    A) 4mm

    B) 1mm

    C) 6mm

    D) 2mm

    E) 8mm

Question 13

You see a patient with a 10–15mm poorly delineated recurrent facial BCC. Which treatment option is the most appropriate?

    A) Surgical excision with 4mm margin

    B) Surgical excision with 6mm margin

    C) 5 FU

    D) Moh's micrographic surgery

    E) Serial surgical excision

Question 14

Which of the following is true with regard to primary cutaneous malignant melanoma?

    A) Most occur in a pre-existing naevus

    B) Incidence is falling

    C) Melanocytes are only found on the skin

    D) Nodular malignant melanoma is the most common subtype

    E) Xeroderma pigmentosum is a risk factor

Question 15

You receive a histology report back on a patient with malignant melanoma. The report mentions Breslow thickness. Where is Breslow thickness measured from?

A) Stratum lucidum

B) Stratum granulosum

C) Stratum corneum

D) Stratum spinous

E) Stratum basale

Question 16

Which of the following is the most common skin cancer found in renal transplant patients?

A) Basal cell carcinoma

B) Superficial spreading malignant melanoma

C) Squamous cell carcinoma

D) Nodular melanoma

E) Lentigo maligna melanoma

Question 17

With regard to dermoid cysts, which of the following is true?

A) They occur especially at the lateral third of the eyebrow

B) They are more common in the elderly population

C) They are usually acquired

D) They do not contain hair, nails or bone-like material

E) They occur especially at the medial third of the eyebrow

Question 18

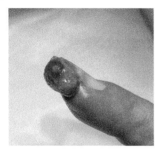

You are asked to see a patient with a lesion on the fingertip. The patient is a seamstress and the lesion started after trauma from a needle a few weeks ago. Which of the following is the most likely diagnosis?

    A) Amelanotic melanoma

    B) Pyogenic granuloma

    C) Exostosis

    D) Squamous cell carcinoma

    E) Digital myxoid cyst

Question 19

Which of the following skin lesions does not have an association with trauma?

    A) Dermatofibroma

    B) Pyogenic granuloma

    C) Keloid

    D) Neuroma

    E) Glomus tumours

Extended Matching Question 20

a) Important differential for pyogenic granuloma

b) Otherwise known as Rodent Ulcer

c) Occurs on the soles and palms most commonly in black and Asian populations

d) Recommended excision margin when excising melanoma in situ

e) Recommended excision margin when excising stage I melanoma

f) Recommended excision margin when excising stage II melanoma

g) Classical edge of a squamous cell carcinoma

h) Most common subtype of melanoma

i) Bowen's disease is a predisposing factor

j) Pigmented nodule with no preceding in-situ phase

A) 2–3mm

B) 5mm

C) 6mm

D) 1.0cm

E) 1.5cm

F) 1–2cm

G) Everted edge

H) Inverted edge

I) Squamous cell carcinoma

J) Basal cell carcinoma

K) Superficial spreading malignant melanoma

L) Nodular melanoma

M) Lentigo maligna melanoma

N) Acral lentiginous melanoma

O) Amelanotic melanoma

Mr Roland Fernandes

FRCS MBBS BSc
General and UGI Surgeon
East Kent Hospital University Foundation Trust

Question 1

The following is true of the inguinal canal except:

A) The conjoint tendon is a fusion of the tranversus muscle and internal oblique muscle

B) Contains the ilioinguinal nerve

C) The internal oblique aponeurosis rolls at its lower edge to form the Poupart's ligament

D) Contains the iliohypogastric nerve

E) Contains the genital branch of the genitofemoral nerve

Question 2

The proportion of patients with an asymptomatic hernia requiring an operation for increasing pain or complications within 5 years is:

A) <1%

B) 5–10%

C) 15%

D) 25%

E) 50%

Question 3

A Kugel repair for inguinal hernia is:

    A) Pre-peritoneal mesh repair

    B) Pre-peritoneal non mesh repair

    C) Repair in which the mesh is sutured in front of the hernia defect anteriorly

    D) Mesh plug repair

    E) Suitable for paediatric inguinal hernias

Question 4

Which of the following is the open equivalent of a laparoscopic TEP Repair?

    A) Bassini

    B) Rives-Stoppa

    C) Shouldice

    D) Kugel

    E) Lichtenstein

Question 5

What is the recurrence rate following an open mesh repair of a unilateral inguinal hernia?

    A) 1%

    B) 2–4%

    C) 7–10%

    D) 10–15%

    E) >15%

Question 6

In ideal mesh should not be:

    A) Lightweight (<80g/m2)

    B) Large pore (>1mm)

    C) Macroporous (>10µm)

    D) Biologically inert

    E) Microporous (<10µm)

Question 7

A 91-year-old frail woman presents with an incarcerated femoral hernia. What surgical access approach would you use?

    A) Low approach (Lockwood)

    B) High approach (McEvedy)

    A) Laparotomy

    B) Palliation

    C) Lotheissen's

Question 8

The following is true of desmoid tumours except:

    A) Have an association with FAP

    B) Can appear in the extremities

    C) Ureteric obstruction can occur as a consequence

    D) Surgical treatment is first line for extra-abdominal desmoids

    E) Anti-testosterone drugs are one of the possible treatment options

Question 9

Which artery passes medial to the femoral ring, along the lacunar ligament and is at risk during femoral hernia repair?

    A) Internal iliac artery

    B) Obturator artery

    C) Inferior epigastric artery

    D) Superior gluteal artery

    E) Inferior gluteal artery

Question 10

Umbilical hernias in children usually resolve by what age?

    A) 3 months

    B) 6 months

    C) 12 months

    D) 24 months

    E) 36 months

Question 11

Which of the following is not a risk factor for a direct inguinal hernia?

    A) Male gender

    B) Cystic fibrosis

    C) High BMI

    D) Collagen vascular disease

    E) Smoking

Extended Matching Question 12

a) Hernia with a hydrocele	A) Spigelian
b) Combined direct and indirect hernia	B) Richter
c) The presence of the appendix within the hernia sac	C) Pantaloon
d) Hernia arising within the transversus abdominis aponeurosis	D) Amyand
e) Femoral hernia in front of the femoral blood vessels	E) Littres
f) Strangulated hernia involving one sidewall of the bowel	F) Velpeau
g) Femoral hernia behind the femoral vessels	G) Gibbon
h) Hernia containing Meckels Diverticulum	H) Narath

CHAPTER 3
HAEMATOLOGY

Answers on page 205–212

Dr Izabela James
Haematology Specialty Trainee and Senior Research Fellow in
Non-Malignant Haematology
Southampton General Hospital, Wessex Deanery

Dr Karan Rangarajan
General Surgery Specialty Trainee
Frimley Park Hospital, Kent Surrey and Sussex Deanery

Question 1

A 68-year-old patient attends pre-op. assessment for elective
laparoscopic cholecystectomy. There is no personal or family
bleeding history and he does not take any medications. He
underwent previous knee replacement without any complications.
Routine clotting screen is done and shows prolonged APTT, which
corrects on mixing studies and subsequent factor levels reveal low
factor XII at 30%. What would you do with this patient?

A) Cancel surgery
B) Treat with FFP preoperatively
C) Treat with cryoprecipitate preoperatively
D) Treat with prothrombin complex concentrate (Octaplex/
   Beriplex) preoperatively
E) Proceed with surgery without any haemostatic cover

Question 2

A 56-year-old patient is planned for an open left inguinal hernia repair. He is on Rivaroxaban for atrial fibrillation. His other past medical history includes hypertension only which is well controlled. His renal function shows CrCl 60ml/min. What is the best management regarding his anticoagulation?

- A) Proceed with surgery without stopping Rivaroxaban
- B) Stop Rivaroxaban 24 hours pre procedure
- C) Stop Rivaroxaban 48 hours pre procedure
- D) Stop Rivaroxaban 72 hours pre procedure
- E) Stop Rivaroxaban 24 hours pre procedure and bridge with LMWH

Question 3

Provided the above operation went uneventfully with no haemostatic issues, anticoagulation with Rivaroxaban can be restarted:

- A) 6 hours post surgery
- B) 12 hours post surgery
- C) 24 hours post surgery
- D) 36 hours post surgery
- E) 72 hours post surgery

Question 4

A 47-year-old builder fell off a ladder at work and sustained significant head injury. He was brought into ED by ambulance, GCS 14/15 (confused). He is on Dabigatran for DVT diagnosed 6 months ago. What is the best management regarding Dabigatran?

- A) Reverse with PCC (prothrombin complex concentrate) only if CT head confirmed intracranial bleed
- B) Reverse with PCC without waiting for the result of CT head
- C) Reverse with FFP without waiting for the result of CT head
- D) Reverse with Idarucizumab (Praxbind) only if CT head confirms intracranial bleed
- E) Reverse with Idarucizumab (Praxbind) without waiting for the result of CT head

Question 5

A 45-year-old man presents to your elective operating list for a reversal of ileostomy. He has a family history of haemophilia and has been diagnosed with mild haemophilia A. Previously he has received repeated transfusions of blood products and factor VIII. Blood tests show [reference values in brackets]:

Haemoglobin: 108 g/L [120–180 g/L],
Prothrombin time (PT): 13 seconds [12–14],
International Normalised Ratio (INR): 1 [0.8–1.1],
Activated partial thromboplastin time (APTT): 55 seconds [28–39],
Factor VIII levels: 15 U/dl [50–150 U/dl].

Choose the true statement regarding the perioperative plan:

A) Only pre-operative restoration of factor VIII levels is likely to be sufficient

B) To manage bleeding, FFP is likely to be administered.

C) Recombinant activated factor VIIa (rFVIIa) would be contraindicated

D) Cover with Tranexamic acid only is unlikely to be sufficient

E) As it is mild heamophilia, bleeding risk due to surgery is very low

Question 6

Chose the most appropriate statement regarding the mode of action of direct oral anticoagulants:

A) Apixaban is a direct thrombin inhibitor, Dabigatran is a direct Xa inhibitor

B) Rivaroxaban is a direct thrombin inhibitor, Dabigatran is direct Xa inhibitor

C) Edoxaban is a direct Xa inhibitor, Dabigatran is a direct thrombin inhibitor

D) Rivaroxaban is a direct Xa inhibitor, Dabigatran is a direct Xa inhibitor

E) Apixaban is a direct Xa inhibitor, Dabigatran is a direct antithrombin inhibitor

Question 7

After routine pre-operative assessment, the haematology laboratory alerts you that it has identified strong cold agglutinin on full blood count. In which type of surgery would a cold agglutinin finding be a contraindication to proceed?

A) Right hemicolectomy

B) Coronary artery bypass graft with cold cardioplegia

C) Dental extraction

D) Cholecystectomy

E) Cataract surgery

Question 8

What minimum platelet count would be safe to proceed with laparoscopic cholecystectomy?

A) 40

B) 50

C) 75

D) 80

E) 100

Question 9

Which is the least likely contributing factor to arterial thrombosis?

A) Diabetes mellitus

B) Smoking

C) Antiphospholipid syndrome

D) Prothrombin gene mutation

E) Hypertension

Question 10

A 75-year-old male is diagnosed with DVT post total sigmoid colectomy. He has impaired renal function with CrCl 35ml/min. His APTR was slightly raised at routine pre-op. assessment and after discussion with haematology lupus anticoagulant screen was done which came back positive. What would be the most appropriate anticoagulant choice for this patient?

A) LMWH followed by Warfarin

B) Dabigatran

C) Rivaroxaban

D) Apixaban

E) LMWH

Question 11

A 52-year-old school teacher is being seen in pre-op. assessment clinic prior to umbilical hernia repair with mesh. He is a non-smoker and does not drink alcohol. He appears well hydrated. He does not take any regular medications apart from occasional paracetamol for headaches. The FBC is as follows:

Hb 193 g/dL
WCC 11.7 x 10E9/L
Neutrophills 10.0 x10E9/L
Platelets 405 x10E9/L
PCV 0.6

What is the most likely haematological diagnosis?

A) Primary polycythaemia

B) Secondary polycythaemia

C) Pseudopolycythaemia

D) Essential thrombocythaemia

E) Myelofibrosis

Question 12

An 82-year-old male patient has been referred to you with abdominal pain and jaundice. On examination, he has widespread low volume cervical, axillary and inguinal lymphadenopathy. He also appears to have splenomegaly palpable 5cm below costal margin. He mentions to you that he has been feeling more tired over the last few days and gets short of breath on minimal exertion. His blood results are as follows:

Hb 75 g/L
WCC 24.1 x 10E9/L
Neutrophils 2.0 x 10E9/L
Lymphocytes 20.4 x 10E9/L

Platelets 280 x 10E9/L
MCV 106 fl
Bilirubin 38 umol/L
ALT 22 U/L

What is the most likely cause of the anaemia?

A) Iron deficiency

B) Autoimmune haemolytic anaemia

C) Anaemia of chronic disease

D) Megaloblastic anaemia

E) Myelofibrosis

Question 13

What further investigations would be most appropriate to confirm the diagnosis?

A) Full iron studies

B) B12 and folate

C) JAK2 mutation analysis

D) Reticulocytes, direct antiglobulin test, haptoglobin, LDH, blood film

E) Bone marrow biopsy

Question 14

Splenomegaly is least likely to be found in:

A) Splenic marginal zone lymphoma

B) Hairy cell leukaemia

C) Chronic lymphoid leukaemia

D) Myelodysplasia

E) Leishmaniasis

Question 15

Which haematological diagnosis warrants need for irradiated blood products irrespective of treatment?

A) Acute myeloid leukaemia

B) Acute lymphoblastic leukaemia

C) Hodgkin lymphoma

D) Follicular lymphoma

E) Mantle cell lymphoma

Question 16

Choose the false statement about Hodgkin lymphoma:

A) There is considerable evidence linking EBV to Hodgkin lymphoma

B) There are four histological subtypes of classical Hodgkin lymphoma: nodular sclerosing, mixed cellularity, lymphocyte depleted, lymphocyte rich

C) Reed Sternberg cells make up only 1–2% of the cellularity of the lymph node

D) Usually presents with painful enlarged cervical lymphadenopathy

E) Bulky mediastinal mass may cause SVC compression

Question 17

The management of the following conditions may include elective splenectomy except:

A) Evans syndrome

B) Autoimmune haemolytic anaemia (AIHA)

C) Hereditary spherocytosis

D) Lymphoma

E) Congenital thrombotic thrombocytopenic purpura (TTP)

Question 18

A 28-year-old patient was diagnosed with Hodgkin lymphoma on cervical lymph node biopsy. There was no history of weight loss or sweats. CT neck/chest/abdomen/pelvis was performed that showed left-sided, superior mediastinal mass measuring 12 x 7.5cm and bilateral supraclavicular fossa lymphadenopathy. The spleen was not enlarged and there were no enlarged abdominal, pelvic or retroperitoneal nodes. What is the Ann Arbor staging of the disease?

A) IA

B) IIA

C) IIB

D) IIS

E) IIIA

Question 19

A 34-year-old male was admitted post road traffic accident. He required surgical intervention and multiple blood products including RBC, FFP and platelets. Few days later he was given 3 units FFP due to deranged clotting prior to central line change. 2 hours after the infusion of FFP he complained of increased shortness of breath and developed cough productive of frothy pink sputum. His oxygen saturation dropped to 87% on air, he became hypotensive with BP 90/65 and had mildly raised temperature 37.6C. You ordered CXR which showed bilateral nodular shadowing and normal heart size. Which of the following is the most likely diagnosis?

A) Transfusion related acute lung injury (TRALI)

B) Transfusion associated circulatory overload (TACO)

C) Acute haemolytic transfusion reaction

D) Febrile non haemolytic transfusion reaction

E) Allergic reaction

Question 20

A 23-year-old female, generally fit and well, originally from Cyprus, has a blood test done prior to abdominoplasty. Her results come back as follows:

Hb 110 g/dL
WCC 6.0 x 10E9/L
Platelets 310 x 10E9/L
MCV 63 fl (77–95 fl)
MCH 19pg (27–32 pg)

Blood film commented on prominent target cells. What is the most likely cause of her anaemia?

    A) Iron deficiency anaemia
    B) βeta thalassaemia major
    C) βeta thalassaemia trait
    D) Sickle cell anaemia
    E) Megaloblastic anaemia

Question 21

What further test would be most useful to confirm diagnosis?

    A) Ferritin
    B) Sickle solubility test
    C) B12 and folate
    D) High-performance liquid chromatography (HPLC)
    E) Reticulocytes

Question 22

A 48-year-old female was admitted electively for Nissens fundoplication. She has metallic mitral prosthesis and therefore was started on unfractionated heparin infusion 24 hours prior to surgery and continued post op. On day 6 post surgery she complained of a painful, swollen left calf. Doppler USS confirmed DVT. She received Vancomycin peri-operatively. Her FBC on day 6 post surgery was as follows:

HB 111 g/L
WCC 12.8 x 10E9/L
Platelets 38 x 10E9/L
Neutrophils 8.7 x10E9/L

What is the most likely diagnosis?

- A) Immune thrombocytopenia
- B) Heparin induced thrombocytopenia (HIT)
- C) Thrombocytopenia secondary to Vancomycin
- D) Thrombotic thrombocytopenic purpura
- E) Disseminated intravascular coagulation (DIC)

Question 23

Choose the false statement regarding neutropenia:

- A) Post infectious neutropenia (most usually post viral) usually resolves within few days of the infection
- B) There is racial variation in neutrophil count – in black and Middle Eastern people mild neutropenia may be normal
- C) Neutropenia is a part of diagnostic criteria in Felty's syndrome
- D) Multiple drugs can cause neutropenia, these include: Phenytoin, Carbimazole, Co-trimoxazole
- E) Neutropenia may be a sign of bone-marrow infiltration with malignant cells

CHAPTER 4
GENETIC ASPECTS OF SURGICAL DISEASE

Answers on page 212–216

Dr Katie Snape
BSc (hons) MBBS MRCP PhD FHEA
Consultant Cancer Geneticist
Southwest Thames Regional Genetics Service
St George's University Hospitals NHS Foundation Trust and St George's University of London

Question 1

This is the pedigree of a family with hyperparathyroidism and hypercalcaemia.

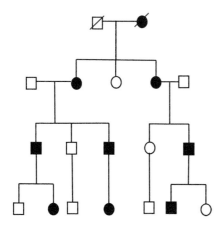

What is the most likely inheritance pattern?

A) Autosomal recessive

B) Autosomal dominant

C) X-linked recessive

D) X-linked dominant

E) Mitochondrial

Question 2

A male patient presents at age 22 with hyperparathyroidism and hypercalcaemia. He tells you that his father had a phaeochromocytoma at age 45 and his paternal grandmother died of thyroid cancer aged 47. What is the most likely genetic diagnosis?

    A) Hereditary phaeochromocytoma-paraganglioma syndrome

    B) Birt-Hogg-Dube syndrome

    C) Multiple endocrine neoplasia type 1

    D) Multiple endocrine neoplasia type 2

    E) Familial hypercalciuric hypercalcaemia (FHH)

Question 3

NICE guidelines recommend offering genetic testing of the high-risk breast and ovarian cancer genes, BRCA1 and BRCA2, when the chance of identifying a mutation is:

    A) 1%

    B) 5%

    C) 10%

    D) 15%

    E) 20%

Question 4

A 39-year-old female presents to the breast clinic with a lump. On investigation this proves to be a benign adenoma. However, she gives a history of her mother having breast cancer aged 53 and her maternal grandmother having breast cancer aged 65. What is the most likely reason for the multiple cases of breast cancer in this family?

    A) BRCA1 mutation

    B) BRCA2 mutation

    C) TP53 mutation

    D) PTEN mutation

    E) Multifactorial inheritance

Question 5

Mutations in which gene cause hereditary diffuse gastric cancer?

A) STK11

B) CDH1

C) PTEN

D) APC

E) MSH2

Question 6

For which of the following conditions would genetic testing be recommended under the age of 5?

A) Lynch syndrome

B) BRCA related breast and ovarian cancer

C) Multiple endocrine neoplasia type 2

D) Hereditary diffuse gastric cancer

E) Multiple endocrine neoplasia type 1

Question 7

A patient presents at age 31 with 60 tubulovillous adenomas in the bowel. Her daughter has just been diagnosed with a hepatoblastoma aged 3. What is the most likely diagnosis?

A) Polymerase "proof reading" polyposis syndrome (PPAP)

B) MUTYH related polyposis

C) Familial adenomatous polyposis

D) Cowden syndrome

E) Peutz–Jeghers syndrome

Question 8

Which of the following patients would be offered a diagnostic genetic test of BRCA1 and BRCA2?

    A) A 60-year-old with high grade serous ovarian cancer, no relevant family history

    B) A 38-year-old with oestrogen positive breast cancer, no relevant family history

    C) A 50-year-old with oestrogen positive breast cancer and a maternal aunt with oestrogen positive breast cancer aged 55

    D) A 70-year-old with a triple negative breast cancer, no relevant family history

    E) A 57-year-old with a mucinous ovarian cancer and a sister with oestrogen positive breast cancer aged 62

Question 9

Which of the following patients would be offered genetic testing for Von Hippel Lindau syndrome?

    A) A 56-year-old male with clear cell renal carcinoma

    B) A 45-year-old female with a secretory pancreatic neuroendocrine tumour (PNET)

    C) A 34-year-old male with hyperparathyroidism

    D) A 39-year-old male with a cerebellar haemangioblastoma

    E) A 61-year-old female with phaeochromocytoma

Question 10

Which of the following patients have an increased risk of endometrial cancer, and risk reducing hysterectomy should be considered?

    A) A female BRCA mutation carrier

    B) A female MLH1 mutation carrier

    C) A female with Peutz–Jeghers syndrome

    D) A female RET mutation carrier

    E) A female with Von Hippel Lindau syndrome

Extended Matching Question 11

A) Lynch syndrome

B) Familial adenomatous polyposis

C) Peutz–Jeghers syndrome

D) Cowden syndrome

E) Hyperplastic/Serrated polyposis syndrome

F) Birt-Hogg-Dube syndrome

G) Hereditary Diffuse Gastric cancer syndrome

H) Polymerase "proof reading" polyposis syndrome (PPAP)

1) Can be identified by undertaking microsatellite instability testing on surgically resected tumour

2) Is also associated with lobular breast cancer

3) Is classically associated with harmatomatous bowel polyps

4) Can be associated with oromucosal hyperpigmentation

5) Is due to mutations in the POLD1/POLE genes

Extended Matching Question 12

A) Daily low-dose aspirin ☐

B) Daily tamoxifen ☐

C) Bilateral risk-reducing mastectomies ☐

D) Risk-reducing total abdominal hysterectomy and bilateral salpingo-oophorectomy ☐

E) Risk-reducing bilateral salpingo-oophorectomy ☐

F) Risk-reducing colectomy ☐

G) Risk-reducing thyroidectomy ☐

H) Whole-body MRI screening ☐

Which of the above would be the most appropriate cancer-risk-management plan to offer to the patients below?

1) A 50-year-old female patient who has two first-degree relatives who both developed bowel cancer in their 50s where investigations for Lynch syndrome are negative in both affected relatives

2) A 45-year-old female patient with Lynch syndrome due to an MSH6 mutation

3) An 18-year-old female patient with Cowden syndrome

4) A 31-year-old female with a BRCA1 mutation

5) A 25-year-old female with an APC mutation

Extended Matching Question 13

A) Medullary thyroid cancer ☐

B) Triple negative breast cancer ☐

C) Colorectal cancer ☐

D) Paraganglioma ☐

E) Retinal angioma ☐

F) Dysplastic gangliocytoma of the cerebellum ☐

G) Basal cell carcinoma ☐

H) Melanoma ☐

Which cancer is most strongly associated with the following genes?

1) BRCA1

2) PTEN

3) VHL

4) PTCH1

5) SDHB

CHAPTER 5
ONCOLOGY FOR SURGEONS

Answers on page 216–218

Mr Roland Fernandes
FRCS MBBS BSc
General and UGI Surgeon
East Kent Hospital University Foundation Trust

Dr Lucy O'Reilly
MBBS BSc
East Kent Hospital University Foundation Trust

Question 1

Which genetic condition is associated with an increased risk of papillary thyroid cancer?

- A) Peutz–Jeghers syndrome
- B) Neurofibromatosis
- C) Familial adenomatous polyposis coli
- D) Multiple endocrine neoplasia type I
- E) Lynch syndrome

Question 2

Obesity increases the risk of malignancy in:

- A) Breast Cancer
- B) Myeloma
- C) Pancreatic cancer
- D) Renal cancer
- E) All of the above

Question 3

The most serious recognised side effect of anthracyclines is:

A) Renal failure

B) Diarrhoea

C) Vomiting

D) Cardiomyopathy

E) Alopecia

Question 4

The mode of action of Imatinib is:

A) Inhibitor of bcr-Abl tyrosine kinase inhibitor

B) Multi-targeted tyrosine kinase inhibitor

C) Topoisomerase II inhibitor

D) Inhibits DNA synthesis

E) Alkylating agent

Question 5

Cyclophosphamide is part of what group of chemotherapy agents?

A) Anti-metabolite

B) Alkylating agent

C) Anti-microtubule agents

D) Topoisomerase II inhibitor

E) Anti-tumour antibiotic

Question 6

Capecitabine is converted by the body to which agent?

A) Folinic acid

B) Cisplatin

C) Cyclophosphamide

D) Gemcitabine

E) 5 – Fluorouracil

Question 7

Which therapeutic agent is correctly matched with its molecular target?

    A) Gefitinib and ERBB2

    B) Imatinib and VEGFR2

    C) Trastuzumab and HER2

    D) Rituximab and proteasome

    E) Lapatinib and ERBB1

Question 8

Herceptin is usually given in early HER positive breast cancer for which duration?

    A) 3 months

    B) 6 months

    C) 1 year

    D) 3 years

    E) 5 years

Question 9

In colorectal cancer a CEA level may be useful in all of the scenarios except:

    A) Prognosis

    B) Following treatment response

    C) Early diagnosis

    D) Identifying recurrence

    E) Two of the above

Question 10

When a patient has a partial response to chemotherapy, this implies what degree of reduction in tumour volume?

    A) At least 10%

    B) At least 20%

    C) At least 30%

    D) At least 40%

    E) At least 50%

Question 11

In the MAGIC trial (2006) looking at adenocarcinoma of oesophagus, GOJ or stomach what chemotherapy regimen was used?

    A) Pre-op FEC (5FU + Epirubicin + Cisplatin)

    B) Peri-operative 5FU + Epirubicin + Cisplatin

    C) Post operative 5FU + Epirubicin + Cisplatin

    D) Peri-operative 5FU + Epirubicin + Cisplatin + radiotherapy

    E) Post operative 5FU + Epirubicin + Cisplatin + radiotherapy

Question 12

In the FLOT trial, what form of cancers were investigated?

    A) Gastric or gastro-oesophageal cancers

    B) Gastric cancers

    C) Oesophageal cancers

    D) Rectal cancers

    E) Pancreatic cancers

Question 13

In the original Heald paper, the local recurrence rates following a TME dissection were reported as:

    A) <30%

    B) <20%

    C) <15%

    D) <10%

    E) <5%

Question 14

The Mercury Trial concerns:

    A) The use of endoanal USS in imaging low rectal cancers

    B) The use of MRI in staging rectal cancers

    C) The use of PET in staging oesophageal cancers

    D) Staging laparoscopy in gastric cancers

    E) CT colonography in colorectal cancer detection

Question 15

What treatment regimen is most common for resectable colorectal liver metastases?

    A) Surgery and adjuvant FOLFOX/FOLFIRI

    B) Chemoradiotherapy

    C) Surgery alone

    D) Neoadjuvant FOLFOX/FOLFIRI followed by surgery and adjuvant chemotherapy

    E) Neoadjuvant FOLFOX/FOLFIRI followed by surgery

Question 16

The following are all contraindications for resection of colorectal liver metastases except?

    A) Recurrence following a first resection

    B) Unresectable extrahepatic disease

    C) Extensive nodal disease

    D) Resection would yield too small a future liver remnant

    E) Unfit for surgery

Question 17

The following are all treatment modalities used in anal SCC except?

    A) Abdominoperineal excision

    B) External beam radiation

    C) Brachytherapy

    D) Chemotherapy

    E) Antiviral therapy

Extended Matching Question 18

A) Cyclophosphamide

B) Hand and foot Syndrome

C) Methotrexate

D) Red urine

E) Purine antagonist

F) Green urine

G) Pyrimidine antagonist

H) Etoposide

I) Anthracycline

J) Peripheral neuropathy

K) Irinotecan

L) Alkylating agent

M) Bleomycin

1) Folate antagonist (metho)

2) Chemotherapy agent known for causing pulmonary fibrosis (Bleo)

3) Topoisomerase I Inhibitor (Etop)

4) Side effect of capecitabine (HFS)

5) Side effect caused by taxanes, vinca alkaloids and platinum agents (PN)

6) Side effect from doxorubicin (red urine)

7) Azathioprine belongs to this class of drug (Purine)

8) 5-fluorouracil belongs to this class of drug (pyrimdine)

CHAPTER 6
PATHOPHYSIOLOGY OF SHOCK AND PERITONITIS

Answers on page 219–223

Dr James Cook
MBBS MSc
Anaesthetics and Intensive Care Registrar
Maidstone and Tunbridge Wells Hospital

Question 1

An elderly man presents to the emergency department acutely unwell with reduced Glasgow Coma Score and abdominal distension. A CT chest and abdomen demonstrates small bowel obstruction and evidence of aspiration. A diagnosis of sepsis is made.

Which of the following physiological markers is no longer needed for the diagnosis of sepsis or septic shock?

    A) Systolic blood pressure less than or equal to 100 mmHg

    B) Altered mental state (GCS <15)

    C) Lactate greater of equal to 2 mmol/L

    D) T >38°C or <36°C

    E) Respiratory rate greater than or equal to 22

Question 2

This patient has not responded to fluid resuscitation and the intensive care registrar would like to admit them to the intensive care unit for blood pressure support. Which inotrope/vasopressor are they likely to start?

A) Dopamine

B) Enoximone

C) Noradrenaline

D) Dobutamine

E) Milrinone

Question 3

A patient post laparotomy has developed acute kidney injury. Which of the following is the strongest indication for admission to intensive care for haemofiltration?

A) Anuria for 6 hours

B) Creatinine >1,000

C) Unable to pass a urinary catheter

D) Oliguria <0.2mls/kg for 12 hours

E) Potassium >6.0 after medical management

Question 4

All of the following shift the oxygen dissociation curve to the right EXCEPT:

A) Increased pCO_2

B) Increased temperature

C) Increased [H+]

D) Increased 2,3 DPG

E) Increased pH

Question 5

A 42-year-old man underwent an elective splenectomy for haematological malignancy 6 months ago. He now presents with overwhelming post-splenectomy infection syndrome (OPSI). Which is the most likely causative organism?

A) *Streptococcus pneumoniae*

B) *Haemophilus influenzae*

C) *Neisseria meningitides*

D) *Escherichia coli*

E) *Pseudomonas aeruginosa*

Question 6

You are asked to see a 22-year-old female who is complaining of acute shortness of breath and chest pain. She has recently had an ankle ORIF and has been reluctant to engage with the physiotherapists due to pain. She has no other medical conditions and her only regular medication is the oral contraceptive pill. Which test is the most specific for the likely cause of her symptoms?

A) Arterial blood gas analysis

B) Chest X-ray

C) D-dimer blood test

D) Computed tomography pulmonary angiography

E) V/Q perfusion scan

Question 7

Physiological effects of pneumoperitoneum during laparoscopic surgery include all of the following EXCEPT?

A) Decreased ICP

B) Reduced venous return

C) Increased airway pressure

D) Reduced functional residual capacity

E) Bradycardia

Question 8

Your anaesthetic colleague plans to site an epidural catheter for post laparotomy analgesia. At what spinal level are they likely to insert the catheter?

A) C6/C7

B) T3/T4

C) T9/T10

D) L3/L4

E) T12/L1

Question 9

A 60 year old with gall stone pancreatitis developed respiratory distress and deteriorated on the ward, requiring intubation and ventilation. Investigations demonstrated bilateral opacities on CXR, a PaO2/FiO2 ratio of <300mmHg, and normal cardiac function on echocardiography. What is the cause of her deterioration?

A) Bilateral pleural effusions

B) Pulmonary atelectasis

C) Aspiration pneumonitis

D) Acute respiratory distress syndrome (ARDS)

E) Pulmonary oedema

Question 10

Which statement is false regarding fluid resuscitation with 1L of fluid?

A) 0.9% saline is isotonic

B) Extracellular fluid accounts for two-thirds of total body water (TBW)

C) If 0.9% saline, 250mls will remain in the intravascular compartment

D) If 5% dextrose, 84mls will remain in the intravascular compartment

E) 60% of an adult male's total body weight is water

Question 11

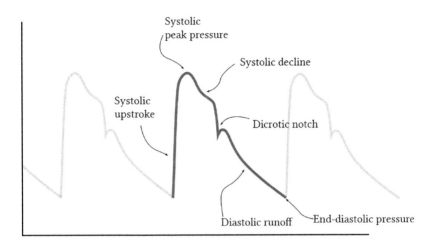

The anaesthetist inserts an arterial line for your patient. What information **cannot** be derived from the arterial line waveform?

    A) Left ventricular contractility

    B) Stroke volume

    C) Peripheral vascular resistance

    D) Fluid responsiveness

    E) Ejection fraction

Question 12

You are operating on a 70kg man who is having an open appendicectomy. The anaesthetist asks if you can infiltrate local anaesthetic into the wound. Which is the most appropriate?

    A) 28 mls 0.5% bupivacaine

    B) 35 mls 0.5% bupivacaine

    C) 25 mls 1% ropivacaine

    D) 28 mls 1% lignocaine

    E) 25 mls 1% lignocaine

Question 13

Your patient underwent a femoral nail operation this morning. The patient is unwell and has been reviewed by the anaesthetist, who calls you to say they feel the patient may have suffered a fat embolism. What is the least likely feature of a fat embolism?

A) Hypoxia

B) Petechial rash

C) Decreased conscious level

D) Photophobia

E) ARDS

Question 14

During an AAA repair, you place an infra-renal cross-clamp. Which physiological change will occur immediately after application of the clamp?

A) Increased heart rate

B) Decreased cardiac output

C) Increased systemic vascular resistance

D) Decreased blood pressure

E) Increased central venous pressure

Question 15

Which of these is NOT a clinical consequence of perioperative hypothermia?

A) Hypotension

B) Tachycardia

C) Reduced oxygen delivery

D) Hyperglycaemia

E) Prolongation of anaesthetic drugs

Question 16

Which of these is a known risk factor for post-op nausea and vomiting?

    A) Smoker

    B) Male

    C) Laparotomy

    D) Regional anaesthesia

    E) Bariatric surgery

Question 17

With regards to re-feeding syndrome, which is incorrect?

    A) Occurs within 72 hours of starting to feed

    B) Sudden rise in insulin secretion

    C) Increased serum levels of phosphate, potassium and magnesium

    D) Shift from fat to carbohydrate metabolism

    E) Decreased serum glucose

Question 18

Which is an equivalent dose to 10mg of oral morphine?

    A) 50mg codeine

    B) 150mg tramadol

    C) 5mg oxycodone

    D) 100mcg fentanyl

    E) 80mg codeine

Extended Matching Question 19

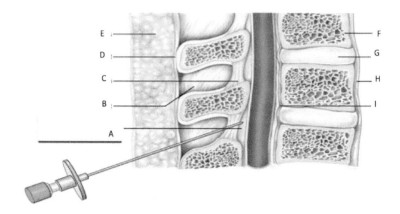

1) Interspinous ligament
2) Intervertebral disk
3) Epidural space
4) Ligametnum flavum
5) Posterior longitudinal ligament
6) Anterior longitudinal ligament
7) Supraspinous ligament
8) Superficial tissue
9) Vertebral body

Extended Matching Question 20

A) Chromaffin cells	1) Secreted from Zona reticularis
B) Aldosterone	2) Stimulates the secretion of cortisol
C) Androgens	3) Catecholamines are synthesised here
D) Zona glomerulosa	4) Outermost zone of adrenal cortex
E) Cortisol	5) Adrenal medulla is stimulated by...
F) ACTH	6) Adrenal cortex is stimulated by...
G) Adrenal medulla	7) Increases the reabsorption of sodium in distal convoluted tubule
H) Sympathetic nervous system	8) Pre-cursor to adrenaline
I) Neuroendocrine control	9) Composed of chromaffin cells
J) L-Tyrosine	10) Increases protein catabolism and gluconeogenesis

Extended Matching Question 21

A) ACE inhibitors	1) Alpha blocker
B) Sodium nitroprusside	2) Pure alpha agonist that can be given peripherally
C) Methyldopa	3) May cause an increase in lactate
D) Phenoxybenzamine	4) Can cause refractory hypotension with anaesthesia
E) Beta blockers	5) Cyanide toxicity is a side effect
F) Meteraminol	6) 1st line vasopressor for low BP due to low SVR
G) Noradrenaline	7) Peripheral vasopressor that is both an alpha and beta agonist
H) Ephedrine	8) Historical antihypertensive still used for hypertension in pregnancy
I) Adrenaline	9) Can cause bronchospasm

Mr Roland Fernandes

FRCS MBBS BSc
General and UGI Surgeon
East Kent Hospital University Foundation Trust

Mr David Swain

Senior Dietician
Basingstoke Hospital

Question 1

The ebb phase of trauma is associated with:

- A) Decreased gluconeogenesis
- B) Decreased glycogenolysis
- C) Increased metabolic rate
- D) Increased sympathetic nervous system activity
- E) Increased resting energy expenditure

Question 2

The flow phase of trauma is associated with:

- A) Decreased heat production
- B) Loss of body nitrogen
- C) Decreased breakdown of fat
- D) Decreased resting energy expenditure
- E) Decreased gluconeogenesis

Question 3

The following is a metabolic response to sepsis:

A) Increase in the peripheral uptake of triacylglycerols

B) Increase in nitrogen levels

C) Decrease gluconeogenesis

D) Decrease in glycogenolysis

E) Increase in rate of glucose uptake by peripheral tissues

Question 4

What is the UK recommended daily intake of protein?

A) 0.2g/kg body weight

B) 0.4g/kg body weight

C) 0.6g/kg body weight

D) 0.75g/kg body weight

E) 1.0g/kg body weight

Question 5

Which of the following statements is untrue with regard to resting metabolic expenditure (RME)?

A) Depends on the type of physical work undertaken

B) Represents the energy required for cardiorespiratory function

C) Helps maintain electrochemical gradients across cell membranes

D) Additional energy requirements in severe sepsis can be up to 0.6 x RME

E) Additional energy requirements in massive burns can be up to 1.0 x RME

Question 6

Which of the following sets of vitamins are all fat soluble?

A) A, B6, B12, D, E

B) A, B6, C

C) B12, D, E, K

D) A, C, D, E

E) A, D, E, K

Question 7

Which of the following trace elements are most important for wound healing?

    A) Iron

    B) Zinc

    C) Copper

    D) Selenium

    E) Iodine

Question 8

A patient in prolonged ileus following a laparotomy for bowel obstruction has been started on parenteral nutrition. He develops psychosis. The depletion of which nutrient is the most likely cause?

    A) Magnesium

    B) Thiamine

    C) Phosphate

    D) Potassium

    E) Glucose

Question 9

What is the aetiology of the biochemical changes observed in refeeding syndrome?

    A) Glycaemia causing an insulin surge and fall in glucagon secretion

    B) Hyperlipidaemia altering metabolism

    C) Fatty acid deficiency

    D) Hypophosphataemia altering tissue compartment distribution

    E) Increased cortisol levels

Question 10

Which of the following is not a metabolic complication of parenteral nutrition?

   A) Hyperglycaemia

   B) Hypoglycaemia

   C) Hypoammonaemia

   D) Hypophosphataemia

   E) Elevations in aspartate aminotransferase

Question 11

Complications of short gut syndrome include all of the following except:

   A) Gallstones

   B) Struvite renal calculi

   C) Peptic ulceration

   D) Slurred speech, ataxia and altered affect

   E) Oxalate renal calculi

Extended Matching Question 12

A) Jejunum ☐

B) Sigmoid colectomy ☐

C) Meckels resection ☐

D) 50cm ☐

E) Cholestyramine ☐

F) Right hemicolectomy ☐

G) Oral isotonic solutions ☐

H) Sleeve gastrectomy ☐

I) Duodenum ☐

J) Creon ☐

K) 100cm ☐

L) Ileum ☐

M) Ensures ☐

N) Oral hypertonic solutions ☐

O) Oral hypotonic solutions ☐

P) 200cm ☐

1) What is the region of small bowel with the maximum water absorption? ☐

2) What is the region of small bowel with the maximum sodium absorption? ☐

A patient has undergone an emergency colorectal operation 6 months ago and is suffering from bile salt malabsorption.

3) What was the most likely operation? ☐

4) What agent can be used in this scenario to improve his symptoms? ☐

5) What is the minimum length of residual jejunum required to avoid supplementary fluid and nutrition in a patient with a jejunostomy? ☐

6) Patients with high output jejunostomies should be encouraged to drink large amounts of which type of fluid? ☐

CHAPTER 8
ACUTE GYNAECOLOGICAL DISEASE

Answers on page 226–230

Dr Jean Kikyo Goodman
MA (cantab) MB BChir MRCOG
Specialist Trainee Year 7 Doctor, Obstetrics and Gynaecology, Health Education England – Wessex

SBA
ECTOPIC PREGNANCY

Question 1
Which of the following is the commonest site for an ectopic pregnancy?

- A) Ovary
- B) Cervix
- C) Uterine cornu
- D) Isthmus of the fallopian tube
- E) Ampulla of the fallopian tube

Question 2
Which of the following is NOT a risk factor for ectopic pregnancy?

- A) Recurrent miscarriage
- B) IVF
- C) Previous chlamydial infection
- D) Smoking
- E) Endometriosis

Question 3

Which of the following is NOT an ultrasound finding consistent with ectopic pregnancy?

A) Adnexal mass

B) Double decidual sign

C) Extrauterine gestational sac

D) Intrauterine pseudosac

E) Free fluid within Pouch of Douglas

Question 4

Which of the following would NOT be considered reasonable first line management of an ectopic pregnancy?

A) Open salpingectomy in the presence of contralateral hydrosalpinx

B) Laparoscopic salpingotomy in the presence of contralateral hydrosalpinx

C) Systemic methotrexate in a haemodynamically stable patient whose βhCG is <5000iu/l

D) Expectant management in a patient willing and able to attend follow up where βhCG is declining

E) Laparoscopic/open salpingectomy in a woman with an adnexal mass of 35mm or larger

PID

Question 5

Which of the following is NOT a reasonable differential diagnosis for pelvic inflammatory disease?

A) Endometriosis

B) Appendicitis

C) Ovarian cyst accident .

D) UTI

E) Polycystic ovarian syndrome

Question 6

Which of the following is a suitable regimen for outpatient antibiotic treatment?

A) Im ceftriaxone 500mg single dose + oral doxycycline 100mg BD 14 days + oral metronidazole 400mg BD 14 days

B) Oral ofloxacin 400mg BD + oral metronidazole 400mg BD, both for 10 days

C) Oral cephalexin 500mg TDS and oral metronidazole 400mg TDS, both for 14 days

D) Im ceftriaxone 250mg single dose + oral azithromycin 1g/week for 4 weeks

E) Im ceftriaxone 250mg single dose + oral doxycycline 100mg BD for 10 days + oral metronidazole 400mg TDS for 10 days

Question 7

Regarding surgical management, which of the following is true?

A) Surgery should be offered to all patients diagnosed with PID

B) Ultrasound guided aspiration of pelvic fluid collections is ineffective

C) Laparoscopic adhesiolysis and drainage of pelvic abscess may lead to early resolution

D) Adhesiolysis for perihepatitis is superior to using antibiotic therapy

E) Surgery should only be offered after unsuccessful ultrasound guided aspiration

Question 8

Which of the following features is NOT suggestive of PID?

A) Bilateral lower abdominal pain

B) Post-coital bleeding

C) Abnormal vaginal discharge

D) Superficial dyspareunia

E) Deep dyspareunia

Question 9

Which of the following is not a known causative agent of PID?

    A) Chlamydia trachomatis

    B) Gardnerella vaginalis

    C) Mycoplasma genitalium

    D) Neisseria gonorrhoea

    E) Yeasts

ENDOMETRIOSIS AND PELVIC PAIN

Question 10

Which of the following is NOT a finding at laparoscopy in a woman with endometriosis?

    A) Endometrioma (chocolate cyst)

    B) Dense adhesions obliterating the Pouch of Douglas

    C) Fibrosis and scarring of the uterosacral ligaments

    D) Perihepatic adhesions

    E) Bluish/red/clear vesicular lesions of the peritoneum

Question 11

Which of the following is NOT a physiological cause of pelvic pain?

    A) Functional ovarian cyst

    B) Ovulation

    C) Polycystic ovaries

    D) Dysmenorrhoea

    E) Blunt trauma to the cervix during sexual intercourse

Question 12

What is demonstrated in the image below?

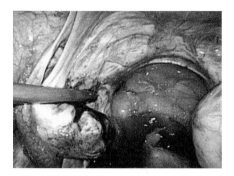

A) Infected pelvic collection

B) Ectopic pregnancy

C) Endometriosis and endometrioma (chocolate cyst)

D) (Ruptured) simple ovarian cyst

E) Retrograde menstruation

OVARIAN MASSES, BENIGN AND MALIGNANT

Question 13

The following are common presenting features of ovarian cancer apart from:

A) Bloating

B) Pelvic pain/pressure

C) Urinary frequency

D) Abnormal vaginal bleeding

E) Loss of appetite

Question 14

Which of the following tumour markers are typically performed in younger women presenting with complex ovarian masses?

A) Ca-125, CEA, Ca-19.9

B) AFP, βhCG, LDH

C) Ca-125, βhCG

D) CEA, AFP, Ca-19.9

E) Ca-125, Ca-15.3, Ca-19.9

Question 15

Which of the following is a classical presentation of ovarian torsion?

A) Cyclical pelvic pain

B) Severe lower abdominal pain associated with vomiting

C) Shock

D) Deep dyspareunia

E) Bilateral severe lower abdominal pain associated with fever (>38°C)

Question 16

Which of the following is the most appropriate management of a simple ovarian cyst of 48mm diameter in a 20 year old?

A) Laparotomy, peritoneal washings and oophorectomy

B) Laparoscopy and oophorectomy

C) Laparoscopy and ovarian cystectomy

D) Antibiotics, analgesia and follow up ultrasound scan in 3 months

E) Analgesia and follow up ultrasound scan in 3 months

Extended Matching Question 17 – Ovarian Cysts

A) Epithelial cell tumours ☐

B) Germ cell tumours ☐

C) Dermoid cysts (mature cystic teratoma) ☐

D) Mucinous type epithelial cell tumours ☐

E) Clear cell carcinoma ☐

F) Krukenberg tumour ☐

G) Theca lutein cysts ☐

H) Brenner Tumours ☐

I) Immature teratomas ☐

J) Lynch I syndrome ☐

K) Lynch II syndrome ☐

From the above, choose the option which best fits the following descriptions:

1) An ovarian cancer with a worse prognosis than other histological types

2) The ovarian tumour which most commonly leads to torsion

3) Type of ovarian cancer more common in afro-caribbean and far eastern ethnicities

4) Bilaterally enlarged ovaries with signet cells on microscopy, associated with metastatic gastric cancer

5) Associated with states of marked βhCG elevation, e.g. in gestational trophoblastic disease

6) Most common ovarian cancer in the first 2 decades of life

7) Associated with pseudomyxoma peritoneii

8) HNPCC syndrome associated with ovarian and endometrial cancer

Extended Matching Question 18 – Pelvic Anatomy – Support of Pelvic Organs

A) Round ligament ☐

B) Broad ligament ☐

C) Cardinal ligament ☐

D) Infundibulopelvic ligament ☐

E) Uterosacral ligament ☐

F) Ovarian ligament ☐

G) Mesosalpinx ☐

H) Pubocervical ligament ☐

I) Urogenital diaphragm ☐

J) Perineal body ☐

Choose the option above which best fits the description below:

1) Thickened band of pelvic fascia running forwards from the cervix and vagina to the pubic bones, supporting the urethra and bladder

2) Extends laterally from the supravaginal cervix and vaginal vault to the pelvic wall

3) A double fold of peritoneum running from the uterus to the fallopian tube superiorly, pelvic wall laterally and pelvic floor inferiorly

4) A 2-layer fibrous sheath running between the ischiopubic rami, superior to the levator ani and pierced by the urethra and vagina

5) A pyramid shaped fibromuscular mass separating the vulva and vagina from the anal canal

6) Ligaments passing back from the cervix to the S2 vertebra

7) Runs laterally between the layers of the broad ligament from the body of the uterus through the inguinal canal to the labia majora

8) Formed from the lateral border of the broad ligament, contains the ovarian vessels

Extended Matching Question 19 – The Clinical pelvis

A) CT chest/abdomen/pelvis ☐

B) MRI pelvis ☐

C) Transvaginal ultrasound scan with measurement of endometrial thickness ☐

D) Bulbospongiosus and transverse perineal muscles ☐

E) Superficial and deep perineal muscles ☐

F) Pubococcygeus, iliococcygeus, ischiococcygeus ☐

G) Deep perineal muscles and puborectalis ☐

H) Pubovaginalis and puborectalis ☐

I) External anal sphincter ☐

J) Internal anal sphincter ☐

K) Anal mucosa ☐

L) Pelvic splanchnic nerves ☐

M) Genitofemoral nerve ☐

N) Ilioinguinal nerve ☐

O) Pudendal nerve ☐

P) Para-aortic lymph nodes ☐

Q) Superficial inguinal lymph nodes ☐

R) Sacral lymph nodes ☐

S) Crossing of the external iliac artery in the pelvic side wall ☐

T) Crossing of the uterine artery lateral to the cervix ☐

U) At the entrance to the bladder ☐

From the above options, choose the most appropriate for the following:

1) A 3c perineal tear involves this muscle

2) Innervation of the perineum and lower ¼ of the vagina, blocked in regional anaesthesia during childbirth

3) Lymphatic drainage of the ovaries

4) A common site of injury to the ureter during hysterectomy

5) Muscles forming the levator ani

6) An accurate imaging method for ruling out endometrial cancer and the need for biopsy

7) Involuntary spasm of these muscles leads to vaginismus

8) Anorectal incontinence may occur as a consequence of this nerve being damaged during traumatic childbirth

CHAPTER 9
EVIDENCE-BASED MEDICINE AND STATISTICAL ANALYSIS

Answers on page 230–235

Dr Jonathan Temple

Department of Women's & Children's Health, King's College London, London, United Kingdom

Great Ormond Street Institute of Child Health, University College London, London, United Kingdom

Dr Seth Seegobin

Department of Biostatistics, Statistical Science and Innovation, UCB, Slough, United Kingdom

Evidence-based medicine, which describes the conscientious and judicious integration of evidence derived from scientific research into everyday clinical practice, continues to drive significant improvement of the safety and efficacy of clinical decision making and patient outcomes. As such, understanding how to effectively and appropriately interpret, evaluate and utilise scientific data in a diverse range of clinical settings represents, arguably, one of the most important skills that healthcare professionals must acquire throughout their training.

This chapter is intended to test the candidate's knowledge of research terminology, methodology and statistical analysis, as well as their skills in evaluating the quality of scientific research.

Question 1

Which of the following experimental hypotheses can be described as 'directional' hypotheses?

(i) People who smoke cigarettes are more likely to develop lung cancer than those who do not smoke.

(ii) The quality of post-operative care affects patient satisfaction.

(iii) The institution of total parenteral nutrition is significantly associated with post-operative morbidity and mortality.

(iv) The incidence of epistaxis in patients on treatment dose enoxaparin is twice as great as in patients on prophylactic dose enoxaparin.

    A) (i) only
    B) (i) and (ii)
    C) (iii) and (iv)
    D) (i) and (iv)
    E) (ii) and (iv)

Question 2

The systematic study of the structure and behaviour of our universe through observation and experimentation forms the foundation of the scientific paradigm, the integrity of which can be said to rest upon several key concepts. Match each each of these concepts to its appropriate definition.

(i) Testability	a) The use of observation and/or experimentation to generate evidence (i.e. information that enables us to verify the degree of truth or falsity of a given proposition)
(ii) Falsifiability	b) The extent to which a proposition can be subjected to robust empirical investigation
(iii) Objectivity	c) The extent to which the findings of an experiment can be considered 'true' or correct
(iv) Empiricism	d) The extent to which a proposition possesses an inherent capacity to be empirically disproved
(v) Validity	e) The extent to which individual bias or belief or external influence upon judgements pertaining to the truth or falsity of a given proposition are absent

Question 3

A surgical registrar conducting an audit into post-operative complications in her department comes to suspect that the introduction of a new suturing material has coincided with a higher incidence of post-operative wound dehiscence. She conducts an experiment that demonstrates the maximum tensile strength of the new suturing material is slightly less than that of other suturing materials already used within the department. She concludes that the lower tensile strength of the new suturing material is directly responsible for the increase in post-operative complications. Which type of experimental bias is this an example of?

    A) Confirmation bias

    B) Attribution bias

    C) Anchoring

    D) Determinism

    E) Statistical bias

Question 4

Only by developing an understanding of the fundamental nature of the various elements within a given experimental system, which are referred to as 'variables', can we begin to attempt to define the relationships that may or may not exist between them and how these relationships might explain the phenomenon being studied. Match each of the following types of variable to its appropriate definition.

(i)	Independent variable	a)	Any element of an experimental system other than the independent variable which can change and therefore affect the dependent variable
(ii)	Extraneous variable	b)	Any element of an experimental system that changes or is expected to change as a direct result of variation in the conditions of the independent variable
(iii)	Control	c)	Any condition of an experiment in which the independent variable is either absent or not directly manipulated by the investigator
(iv)	Dependent variable	d)	Any element of an experimental system other than the independent variable and dependent variable
(v)	Confounding variable	e)	Any element of an experimental system that is directly manipulated by the researcher

Question 5

Healthcare professionals are increasingly required to develop an understanding as to how scientific data should be interpreted, evaluated and utilised in a diverse range of clinical settings. As such, they must first acquire a clear yet comprehensive understanding of the language and terminology of scientific research. Match each of the following terms to its most appropriate definition.

(i) External validity	a) The extent to which the findings of an experiment remain unchanged when that experiment is repeated, under the same experimental conditions
(ii) Generalisability	b) The extent to which events within a given system, including the outcomes of an experimental system, are presented as the inevitable product of chains of causality
(iii) Internal validity	c) The extent to which the findings of a study or experiment can be applied to individuals, groups or situations beyond those that were included within the confines and limitations of the experimental system in which they were obtained
(iv) Replicability	d) The extent to which an experiment has been successful in measuring the effect of the independent variable upon the dependent variable
(v) Determinism	e) The extent to which the experimental design is successful in faithfully recreating the phenomenon being studied

Question 6

Understanding the limitations of a given study also requires us to recognise the limitations of the data upon which the integrity of its conclusions rests and the means by which that data has been gathered. Match each of the following terms to its most appropriate definition.

(i) Specificity	a) The level of consistency of individual measurements within a single condition of an experiment when those measurements are repeated, within an unchanged experimental system
(ii) Accuracy	b) The degree of refinement within a measurement, calculation or specification or, rather, the 'exactness' or detail with which the investigator records measurements, calculations or specifications
(iii) Reliability	c) The extent to which a single measurement, calculation or specification can be said to conform to the 'true value' the investigator is attempting to measure, calculate or specify within an experiment
(iv) Sensitivity	d) The probability that an actual negative finding will be correctly identified when it occurs
(v) Precision	e) The probability that an actual positive finding will be correctly identified when it occurs

Question 7

A Surgical Registrar is investigating the quality of referrals to General Surgery from the Emergency Department, in the hospital in which they work. Their research hypothesis states that "all surgical referrals from the Emergency Department are appropriate". Which of the following statements represents the most appropriate null hypothesis for this study?

A) No surgical referrals from the emergency department are appropriate

B) Not all surgical referrals from the emergency department are appropriate

C) All surgical referrals from the emergency department are inappropriate

D) Some surgical referrals from the emergency department are not appropriate

E) Only some surgical referrals from the emergency department are appropriate

Question 8

A surgical registrar undertakes an audit of departmental compliance with weekend handover sheets, which summarise the clinical details of each patient and their management plans. She tells anyone who asks that she is, instead, only undertaking an audit of the diagnoses of surgical patients. Which of the following ethical considerations is most affected by her decision to conduct her study in this manner?

A) Confidentiality

B) Informed consent

C) Deception

D) Beneficience

E) Justice

Question 9

Experimental data can be either qualitivative or quantitative. Which of the following research questions are most likely to generate qualitative data?

(i)   What proportion of patients who are prescribed antihypertensive medications are non-compliant?

(ii) Which are the most common post-operative complications following laparoscopic cholecystectomy?

(iii) Why are certain patients who are prescribed antihypertensive medications non-compliant?

(iv) What is the impact of stoma formation upon the emotional wellbeing of patients with Inflammatory Bowel Disease?

A) All of them

B) (i) and (ii)

C) (iii) and (iv)

D) (i) and (iv)

E) (i) only

Question 10

Box plots represent an effective means of respresenting groups of numerical data through their quartiles. Match each component of the diagram below to what it represents.

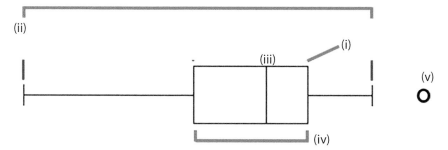

A) The median

B) An outlier

C) Interquartile rank

D) Range

E) First quartile

Question 11

Which of the following definitions encapsulates the meaning of the term '95% confidence interval'?

A) The range of values that one can be 95% certain contains the true mean of the study population

B) The range that encompasses 95% of the sample data values

C) A measure of uncertainty associated with the mean estimate

D) a and c

E) a, b and c

Question 12

Which of the following definitions best encapsulates the meaning of the term 'P Value'?

    A) The probability that the results are clinically relevant

    B) Informs the researcher if the sample size is adequate

    C) The probability of observing the data in the sample given that the alternative hypothesis is true

    D) The probability of observing the data in the sample given that the null hypothesis is true

    E) Equal to 1 minus the confidence interval

Question 13

Which of the following diagrams demonstrates a normal distribution?

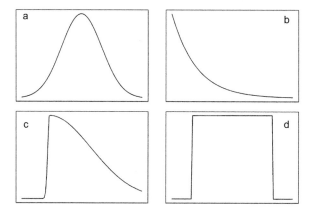

Question 14

Counting Possible Outcomes: A linear arrangement of three deoxyribonucleic acid (DNA) nucleotides is called a triplet. A nucleotide may contain any one of four possible bases: adenine (A), cytosine (C), guanine (G) and thymine (T). How many different triplets are possible?

    A) 4

    B) 12

    C) 32

    D) 64

    E) 128

Question 15

A candidate sitting their exam may receive a grade of high (H), medium (M) or low (L) on a written test, and a grade of either proficient (P) or non-proficient (N) on a practicum. How many different outcomes are there if both tests are taken?

    A) 3

    B) 6

    C) 8

    D) 27

    E) Cannot be calculated without more information

Question 16

The primary objective of a statistical analysis within clinical research is to infer the effectiveness of a treatment to a population of patients by exploring treatment response in a sample of representative patients. Match each statistical test with the most appropriate experimental scenario.

(i) Paired T-Test	a) Investigating the relationship between a surgeon's hours of surgical experience and the incidence of post-operative complications
(ii) Chi-square	b) Comparing the systolic and diastolic blood pressure values of patients with hypertension before and after administration of antihypertensive medication
(iii) Mann-Whitney U Test	c) Comparing the difference in pain scores between men and women with acute appendicitis
(iv) Spearman Correlation	d) Comparing the pain scores of patients with acute abdominal pain before and after review by the acute pain management team
(v) Un-paired T Test	e) Comparing the incidence of flu-like symtoms among surgical inpatients over the age of 60 who either have or have not received their annual flu vaccination

ACKNOWLEDGEMENTS

We would like to acknowledge and thank Ian Bowen, David Wallace, Darren Elliott, Thanesan Ramalingam, Alastair Sutcliffe, Jude A. Oben, Helena Coomber and Magnus Seegobin, without whose encouragement and support this chapter could not have been written.

FURTHER READING

Glasziou, P.P., et al. (2007) *Evidence-Based Practice Workbook*, 2nd Edition. BMJ Books.
Greenhalgh, T. (2014) *How to Read a Paper.*
Motulsky, H. (2010) *Intuitive Biostatistics: A Nonmathematical Guide to Statistical Thinking.* New York, Oxford University Press.
Sackett, D., et al. 'Evidence based medicine: what it is and what it isn't'. *BMJ*, 1996, 312: 71
Zar Jerrold, H. (1996) *Biostatistical Analysis.* Prentice Hall, Upper Saddle River.

Dr Lulia Al-Hillawi

BSc(Hons), MBBS, MRCP(UK)
Gastroenterology Specialist Registrar, Maidstone and Tunbridge Wells NHS Trust

Question 1

Which of the following scoring systems is recommended by NICE and the British Society of Gastroenterology (BSG) as a pre-endoscopy risk stratification tool?

A) CLIF-SOFA score

B) AIMS65

C) Forrest classification

D) Glasgow-Blatchford score

E) Rockall score

Question 2

A 75-year-old man with a background of end-stage renal failure and ischaemic heart disease is admitted with a 2-day history of melaena. He is anticoagulated with apixaban for atrial fibrillation. Observations are as follows: T 36.7 RR18 sats 95% on room air BP 100/60 HR 90. According to the Rockall score, what single feature carries the highest mortality risk for the patient?

A) Anticoagulation with apixaban

B) BP of 100/60

C) End-stage renal failure

D) Ischaemic heart disease

E) Age of 75

Question 3

Given the active bleed, the team decide to reverse the anticoagulant properties of the apixaban. What is the reversal agent for apixaban?

    A) Platelet transfusion

    B) Beriplex 25 IU/kg IV

    C) Fresh frozen plasma (FFP) 10–15ml/kg IV

    D) Vitamin K 10mg IV

    E) None of the above

Question 4

At endoscopy, he is found to have a 2cm ulcer at D1 with a visible vessel in the ulcer base. What is the Forrest classification of this ulcer?

    A) Ia

    B) Ib

    C) IIa

    D) IIb

    E) IIc

Question 5

What is the single best therapy for the patient's duodenal ulcer?

    A) Oral PPI

    B) 72 hours IV PPI infusion

    C) Adrenaline injection and 72 hours IV PPI infusion

    D) Adrenaline injection and clip placement

    E) No treatment indicated

Question 6

A 75-year-old patient has a background of end-stage renal failure and ischaemic heart disease, BP 100/60 HR 90, endoscopy findings of duodenal ulcer with visible vessel. Given the clinical and endoscopic findings, what is his post-endoscopy Rockall score?

    A) 4

    B) 5

    C) 6

    D) 7

    E) 8

Question 7

A 20-year-old patient presents to A&E with a history of syncope and melaena. Her haemoglobin is 120g/l, urea 4.5, creatinine 70. Platelets and coagulation screen are within normal range. She has no relevant past medical history. Medication list includes ibuprofen as required for period pain. Observations: T37, RR16, sats 100% on room air, BP 130/70, HR 60. You work out her Glasgow-Blatchford score as 3 and discuss admission for OGD.

In terms of her Glasgow-Blatchford score, which feature carries more weight in the scoring and thus gives higher risk of requiring intervention?

    A) Haemoglobin of 120g/l

    B) Systolic blood pressure 130mmHg

    C) Presence of melaena

    D) Syncope

    E) Ibuprofen use

Question 8

A 37 year old is admitted with haematemesis. She is hypotensive and tachycardic with reduced conscious level, responding to pain stimuli only. On examination the A&E registrar has noted spider naevi across the chest wall, mild jaundice and palmar erythema. Whilst examining her she has a large volume haematemesis of 500mls. Her blood tests are as follows:

WCC 5.0 Hb 58 platelets 90 MCV 105 Na 128 K 3.5 creat 40 albumin 25 bilirubin 250 ALP 180 ALT 300 INR 2.8

What is the single best intervention proven to improve this patient's mortality?

    A) Urgent OGD+variceal banding

    B) IV terlipressin 2g

    C) IV co-amoxiclav 1.2g

    D) 1 unit RBC transfusion

    E) 10mg IV vitamin K

Question 9

The patient undergoes OGD plus variceal banding to oesophageal varices. She continues to have active haematemesis post-procedure. What is the single best definitive treatment?

A) Repeat OGD + repeat variceal banding

B) Repeat OGD + injection of cyanoacrylate glue

C) Balloon tamponade

D) Laparotomy

E) Transjugular intrahepatic portosystemic shunt

Question 10

According to BSG and NICE guidance, endoscopy for acute upper GI bleeding should be performed within:

a) 1 hour

b) 4 hours

c) 12 hours

d) 24 hours

e) 72 hours

Question 11

A 70-year-old female with past medical history of COPD and previous breast cancer has undergone a second OGD plus endoscopic therapy for a large bleeding ulcer within the duodenal bulb. You are called to review her on the ward due to coffee ground vomiting and a drop in blood pressure. There is further evidence of active bleeding with drop in Hb and active melaena. What is the single best definitive treatment for this lady?

A) Continue IV PPI infusion

B) Continue IV PPI infusion and add tranexamic acid

C) Repeat OGD with further endoscopic therapy

D) Laparoscopic repair with omental patch

E) Transcatheter arterial embolisation of the left gastric artery

Question 12

A 50-year-old gentleman who underwent a total knee replacement 2 weeks previously is admitted with hypovolaemic shock and a 3-day history of melaena. He has been taking naproxen for pain post-operatively and LMWH as VTE prophylaxis. His past medical history is relevant for being a Jehovah's witness. He tells you that he would not accept RBC transfusion under any circumstance and accepts risk of death by refusing. He has a valid Advance Decision with him to this effect. Blood tests reveal a haemoglobin of 55g/l with normal coagulation screen and platelet count. He has a stage 1 AKI. His blood pressure drops further to 70/40 with a heart rate of 110bpm and he becomes more drowsy. His family arrive and his wife begs you to give him a life-saving blood transfusion. She threatens to sue you for negligence. What is the most appropriate course of action?

A) 2 units O negative red blood cell transfusion

B) IV crystalloid and request ITU input for inotropic support

C) Stop all treatment given the patient's prior wishes

D) Do not administer any treatment until consultation with the trust's medicolegal team

E) IV FFP

Extended Matching Question 13

a) No follow up ☐

b) Repeat OGD in 1 day ☐

c) Repeat OGD in 1 week ☐

d) Repeat OGD in 2–4 weeks ☐

e) Repeat OGD in 6–8 weeks ☐

f) Referral for transjugular intrahepatic portosystemic shunt ☐

g) Amoxicillin 1g PO BD, metronidazole 400mg BD for 2 weeks and omeprazole 40mg BD for 4 weeks ☐

h) Amoxicillin 1g PO BD, metronidazole 400mg BD for 2 weeks and omeprazole 40mg BD for 4 weeks followed by repeat OGD to check for ulcer healing ☐

From the above options, match the correct follow-up plan to the following cases of upper GI bleeding:

1) A 3cm gastric ulcer with clean base in the greater curve of the stomach

2) 3x 2cm ulcers with haematin spot in D1 and D2

3) 4 large columns of oesophageal varices, banded at OGD; haemostasis achieved

4) 4 large columns of oesophageal varices, banded at OGD; further haematemesis requiring intubation and Sengstaken tube insertion on day 2

5) Mallory–Weiss tear

Extended Matching Question 14

a) 3 columns of grade 2–3 oesophageal varices with cherry red spot ☐

b) Mallory–Weiss tear ☐

c) 3cm cratered ulcer in the greater curve of the stomach ☐

d) 2cm ulcer in D1 with arterial spurting ☐

e) No evidence active/recent bleeding identified at OGD ☐

f) Portal hypertensive gastropathy with oozing from the mucosa ☐

g) Grade III reflux oesophagitis ☐

h) Large sliding hiatus hernia ☐

From the above options, match the most likely endoscopic diagnosis to the presentation below:

1) 25 year old admitted with fresh haematemesis. He reports violent episodes of vomiting overnight with subsequent small volume haematemesis with clots. He admits to drinking alcohol to excess the night before at a work party.

2) 68-year-old man admitted with syncope and found to have a haemoglobin of 87g/l. He has a past medical history of recently diagnosed gout for which he has been taking naproxen.

3) 15-year-old girl admitted with a fainting episode, with recurrent episodes of abdominal pain and bloody diarrhoea over the last 6 months.

4) 85-year-old inpatient following a stroke, referred due to anaemia and coffee ground vomiting.

5) 42 year old admitted with haematemesis and 3-day history of black tarry stool. His past medical history is significant for obesity and type 2 diabetes mellitus. He is jaundiced on admission with evidence of hypovolaemic shock.

6) 42 year old admitted with haematemesis. His past medical history is significant for chronic hepatitis B. He has stigmata of chronic liver disease. His observations are stable.

Question 15

The Bristish Society of Gastroenterology published guidelines for the management and diagnosis of lower GI bleeding in 2019. What factor is used to classify bleeding patients into stable and unstable?

A) Pulse
B) MAP
C) Hb
D) Shock index
E) Systolic BP

Question 16

For lower GI bleeds that are classified as unstable, what is the most appropriate investigation or treatment following initial resuscitation?

A) CT angiogram
B) Laparotomy
C) On-table colonoscopy and laparotomy
D) Urgent colonoscopy
E) OGD

Question 17

A 76-year-old man with an unstable PR bleed undergoes a CT angiogram that fails to identify the source of bleeding. What is the next most appropriate procedure or investigation?

A) CT angiogram repeated when active bleeding
B) Laparotomy
C) On-table colonoscopy and laparotomy
D) Urgent colonoscopy
E) OGD

Question 18

Stable lower GI bleeding patients are further classified as to major and minor by what criteria?

    A) Blatchford

    B) Oakland

    C) Breslow

    D) Fong

    E) Heger

Question 19

What is the correct management for stable minor risk lower GI bleeding patients?

    A) CT angiogram

    B) Inpatient colonoscopy

    C) Inpatient OGD and flexible sigmoidoscopy

    D) Inpatient flexible sigmoidoscopy

    E) Discharge and outpatient endoscopy

Question 20

What is the correct management for stable major risk lower GI bleeds?

    A) CT angiogram

    B) Inpatient colonoscopy

    C) Inpatient OGD and flexible sigmoidoscopy

    D) Inpatient flexible sigmoidoscopy

    E) Discharge and outpatient endoscopy

Question 21

What is the accepted haemoglobin level at which a blood transfusion is recommended in a patient without cardiovascular disease?

    A) Hb <60g/L

    B) Hb <70g/L

    C) Hb <80g/L

    D) Hb <90g/L

    E) Hb <100g/L

Question 22

A 76-year-old gentleman is known to have coronary stents and is on both aspirin and clopidogrel. He presents with a lower GI bleed and has a pulse of 76 and BP 128/70. His Oakland score is 7. What would you do about his medications?

A) Discontinue both

B) Discontinue aspirin

C) Discontinue clopigrel

D) Discontinue both and replace with LMWH

E) Continue both

Question 23

What is the reversal agent of dabigatran?

A) Prothrombin complex

B) Vitamin K

C) Protamine sulphate

D) Idarucizumab

E) There are no reversal agents available

CHAPTER 11

ABDOMINAL PAIN IN CHILDHOOD

Answers on page 248–251

Miss Katherine Pearson
BMedSci (Hons) BMBS PGCert (MedEd) FRCS
ST8 General Surgical Registrar
University Hospital Southampton

ABDOMINAL PAIN IN CHILDHOOD

Extended Matching Question 1

1) Appendicitis ☐
2) Constipation ☐
3) Urinary tract infection ☐
4) Mesenteric adenitis ☐
5) Intussusception ☐
6) Ectopic pregnancy ☐
7) Ruptured ovarian cyst ☐
8) Crohn's disease ☐

For each of the following scenarios, choose the single most likely diagnosis from the list above. Each option may be used once, more than once or not at all.

a) A 9-year-old girl is brought into hospital by her mother with a 2-day history of right iliac fossa pain. She has had a runny nose for the past few days but is eating and drinking well despite the pain. On examination she is afebrile and tender in the right iliac fossa with some guarding. There is a strong family history of inflammatory bowel disease.

b) A 10-month-old presents with episodes of drawing up of their legs associated with crying and some bloody runny stools.

c) A 3-year-old child presents with his parents with a 24-hour history of fever, vomiting and abdominal pain.

d) A 14-year-old boy presents with 4 weeks of being generally unwell, some vague abdominal pain and diarrhoea up to 10 times a day. His mother says his clothes don't fit him anymore and she thinks he has lost weight.

e) A 15-year-old girl is brought in by ambulance tachycardic and slightly hypotensive with left iliac fossa pain and peritonism.

Question 2

When considering the presentation of possible appendicitis in children, the following are all true except:

A) Delays in presentation to hospital and diagnosis are seen more commonly in children than in adults

B) Frequent repeated examinations are a useful diagnostic aid

C) The classical history of migratory iliac fossa pain is seen more commonly in older rather than younger children

D) An option in the management of an appendix mass is conservative treatment

E) The laparoscopic approach to appendicectomy is inappropriate in children younger than 5 years

INTUSSUSCEPTION

Question 3

The following are true of intussusception except:

A) It most commonly presents at 2 years of age

B) Boys are more frequently affected than girls

C) A 'red currant jelly' stool of blood and mucus is commonly passed

D) Dance's sign may be present

E) In 90% of patients there is no obvious cause

Question 4

Regarding intussusception, please select the incorrect answer:

A) USS is the first line investigation of a patient with suspected intussusception

B) Peritonism at presentation is an indication for surgery as first line treatment

C) Air enema reduction is successful in around 85% of cases

D) Air enema reduction should not be repeated if a first attempt is unsuccessful

E) Recurrence would usually occur within 2–3 days

GROIN AND SCROTAL LUMPS

Extended Matching Question 5

1) Analgesia and careful monitoring ☐
2) Surgical ligation or interventional radiology embolisation ☐
3) Jaboulay procedure ☐
4) Antibiotics ☐
5) Patent processus vaginalis ligation ☐
6) Aspiration ☐
7) Herniotomy ☐
8) Immediate scrotal exploration ☐

For each of the following scenarios, choose the single most appropriate treatment from the list above. Each option may be used once, more than once or not at all.

a) A 4-year-old boy is brought into the hospital by his parents. He has a red, swollen scrotum but is not complaining of any pain. On examination there is no tenderness but the whole of his perineum is red and oedematous.

b) A 3-year-old boy is brought to clinic by his mother with a painless swelling of his right hemi scrotum which she has noticed but doesn't bother the child. It transilluminates with a pen torch.

c) A 15-year-old boy presents with a 4-hour history of a tender, swollen left testicle. He is sexually active.

d) A 10-year-old boy presents with a dragging feeling and asymmetrically swollen left hemi scrotum.

ACUTE SCROTUM

Question 6

An 11-year-old boy presents with a 4-hour history of severe pain in his left scrotum. Which of the following statements is correct?

A) Testicular torsion is the most common cause of an acute scrotum in a child

B) The clinical suspicion of testicular torsion is raised on seeing a blue spot at the upper pole of the testis

C) The risk of testicular torsion is increased in unoperated cryptorchid testes

D) The risk of testicular torsion begins to fall after age 10

E) Scrotal infection is common in pre-pubescent boys

PAEDIATRIC TRAUMA

Question 7

Regarding trauma and its management in children, pick the single correct answer:

A) Trauma is the commonest cause of death in the paediatric population under 1 year of age

B) When considering the airway, an infant should have its head in the flexed position due to the large occiput

C) Intraosseous needle insertion should occur if unable to gain access in 60 seconds

D) Hypotension will occur when 10% of circulatory volume is lost

E) Isolated head injury is unusual in paediatric trauma

Question 8

A 7-year-old child presents having fallen from his bicycle and his abdominal examination reveals bruising and tenderness with guarding across his upper abdomen. He is complaining of ongoing abdominal pain and has vomited a couple of times. An USS shows some free fluid. With regards to the most likely diagnosis, all are true except:

    A) A CT scan should be performed

    B) The condition should be managed conservatively in the majority of cases

    C) It is likely to be an isolated injury

    D) There is a high likelihood of needing tertiary input

    E) Biochemical changes in blood tests may be present

Question 9

In a child presenting with seat-belt bruising on their torso all the following injuries should be considered except:

    A) Thoracic spine fracture

    B) Small bowel injury

    C) Lumbar spine fracture

    D) Splenic laceration

    E) Mesenteric injury

UMBILICAL HERNIAS

Question 10

A one-year-old girl is brought to the outpatient clinic by her mother with an umbilical hernia. Which of the following is true?

    A) The child is likely to have an associated abnormality

    B) Umbilical hernias are largest at birth and decrease in size as the child grows

    C) Umbilical hernias are a common cause of abdominal pain in this age group

    D) This should be fixed before her second birthday

    E) Strangulation is extremely rare

INGUINAL HERNIAS

Question 11

Regarding acute presentation, please select the single incorrect answer

A) A 1-month-old baby who presents with an irreducible inguinal hernia needs immediate transfer to the local paediatric surgical centre

B) Every attempt should be made to reduce the hernia including using IV morphine

C) If reduction is not achieved, then the patient should proceed straight to theatre

D) If reduction is achieved, hernia repair should be booked for between 6 and 12 months of age

E) All babies presenting with an inguinal hernia have an increased risk of a hernia on the contralateral side

TONGUE TIE

Question 12

All the following statements are correct except:

A) Occurs when the lingual frenulum is short and attaches nearer the tip of the tongue

B) Intervention may be required if the tongue cannot protrude beyond the lower lip

C) Older children may present with not being able to lick an ice-cream

D) If intervention is required in a neonate, the tight frenulum should be divided under a general anaesthetic

E) Ongoing issues following division could be secondary to a posterior tongue tie

MECKEL'S DIVERTICULUM

Question 13

Please select the incorrect answer:

A) Is typically found in the ileum

B) Occurs in about 2% of the population

C) In a small proportion of children, the diverticulum is lined with ectopic gastric mucosa

D) Patients usually present with painful bleeding

E) A technetium scan may be used for diagnostic purposes

DUODENAL ATRESIA

Question 14

Please select the incorrect answer:

a) Is associated with Down's syndrome in 30% of cases

b) Oligohydramnios is a diagnostic feature on antenatal ultrasound

c) Babies typically present with acute obstruction

d) A 'double bubble' sign is commonly seen on a plain abdominal radiograph

e) Treatment is by duodeno-duodenostomy

PYLORIC STENOSIS

Question 15

A 4-week-old baby boy is brought to the ED by his parents with projectile, non-bilious vomiting. Please select the correct answer:

A) There is an 80% likelihood of a family history of this condition

B) The baby is likely to be a poor feeder with a lack of hunger

C) Metabolic acidosis is most commonly seen

D) Hypochloraemia, hyponatraemia and hypokalaemia frequently develop

E) Early surgery is important in management of this condition

Question 16

Regarding the investigation and management of the above patient, please select the incorrect answer from the following:

A) Clinical examination may reveal visible peristaltic waves which are secondary to slowly progressive obstruction

B) Palpation of an abdominal mass, typically in the right upper quadrant or epigastrium, is best done with the stomach empty

C) An ultrasound scan is commonly used as a diagnostic aid

D) If the diagnosis is confirmed, a Ladd's procedure should be performed

E) Perforation of the duodenum is a recognised complication of the operative management of this condition

CHAPTER 12
UPPER GASTROINTESTINAL SURGERY

Answers on page 251–262

Mr Sanjay Vasantrao Joshi
MBBS, MS, MSc, FRCSEd, FRCS (UGI)
Associate Specialist UGI Surgery,
Maidstone and Tunbridge Wells NHS Trust
GI SBAs and EMQs

Question 1

A 56-year-old male has reflux symptoms. You see him in clinic and arrange an OGD. This shows the following picture. Which statement is correct in relation to this condition?

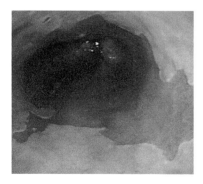

A) It is a common and normal finding

B) It should be biopsied to confirm the diagnosis

C) Presence of intestinal metaplasia in the biopsy sample is a must for diagnosis

D) The patient should have surveillance every 2 years

E) Antireflux surgery is curative procedure for this condition

Extended Matching Question 2 – Barrett's Oesophagus/Early Barrett's Cancer

a) No need to continue surveillance ☐

b) Surveillance every 3–5 years ☐

c) Surveillance every 2–3 years ☐

d) Repeat biopsy at 6 months ☐

e) End of surveillance & refer to MDM ☐

f) EMR (Endoscopic mucosal resection) ☐

g) Radiofrequency ablation ☐

h) OGDs and biopsies at 1 year ☐

i) EUS (endoluminal USS) ☐

j) Two separate pathologists ☐

For each of the following descriptions, choose the single most likely option from the list above. Each option must be used once, more than once or not at all.

1) A 58-year-old man presents on urgent referral pathway with symptoms of dysphagia. An OGD shows a suspicious lesion. The biopsies and further investigations confirm an early intramucosal cancer of oesophagus with stage T1a. His case is discussed in MDM. What is most likely treatment option that will be offered to him?

2) A Barrett's surveillance patient is found to have high grade dysplasia in the biopsies. What will be your next step?

3) A 70-year-old medium-built patient with multiple comorbidities presents with recent onset reflux symptoms. On OGD he is found to have 2cm Barrett's oesophagus confirmed on biopsies with no intestinal metaplasia. He has no family history of cancer of the oesophagus and is a non-smoker. A repeat OGD after 6 months again fails to show intestinal metaplasia in the biopsies. What will be best surveillance advice as per latest BSG guidelines?

4) A 58-year-old woman has reflux symptoms. OGD shows 2cm Barrett's oesophagus with intestinal metaplasia. When should she have surveillance OGD?

5) An elderly patient's Barrett's surveillance OGD shows low-grade dysplasia. You advice high-dose PPI treatment. What will be your next step?

6) An obese 50 year old with long-term GORD symptoms has been found to have 5cm (C3M5) Barrett's oesophagus. How often should he have surveillance OGD?

7) A patient with low-grade dysplasia within a 4cm Barrett's segment is discussed at MDM. There is no visible lesion on repeat OGD and biopsies reconfirm LGD only. What is the most appropriate treatment option for him?

8) A patient is found to have a raised area within Barrett's oesophagus. The biopsies show HGD. What is next treatment that will be offered?

9) What step is mandatory in confirming HGD in Barrett's biopsy samples?

10) A 72-year-old patient on long-term Barrett's surveillance was found to have a suspicious lesion in the lower oesophagus. The biopsy shows this to be early oesophageal cancer spreading to submucosa (T1b). How will you assess the local status of the tumour?

Question 3

A 39-year-old male presents with progressive reflux and dyspepsia. An OGD report shows slightly dilated oesophagus with food debri. The lower sphincter is closed but opens with a pop. Which one of the following statements is correct, given the above description?

A) Patient will benefit from antireflux procedure
B) Biopsy is necessary for the diagnosis of this condition
C) Oesophageal manometry is a gold-standard investigation
D) Long-term treatment options include botox injections
E) Chicago classification differentiates this condition into 2 types

Question 4

Which of the following statements about blood supply to the stomach is correct?

A) Comes from coeliac axis with contribution from superior mesenteric artery

B) Of the 3 branches of coeliac axis, left gastric and hepatic artery supply the stomach while the third branch supplies only spleen

C) Right gastroepiploic artery can be sacrificed during mobilisation of the stomach into chest for Ivor Lewis oesophago-gastrectomy

D) A branch of the right gastric artery contributes to blood supply of lower oesophagus

E) Splenectomy during partial or subtotal gastrectomy can lead to proximal gastric necrosis

Question 5

Which of the gastric lymph-node stations can be left behind during radical (D2) partial gastrectomy for antral gastric cancer?

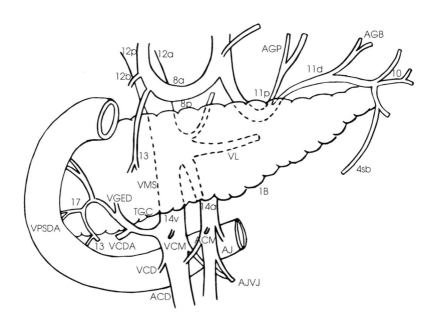

A) 1, 2, 3, 10, 11, 12

B) 1, 2, 4sa, 10, 11, 12

C) 2, 4sa, 10, 11d

D) None – all stations need to be removed

E) Remove what you can

Question 6

A 72-year-old man presents with progressive dysphagia. An OGD shows ulcerated growth at 32cm in mid oesophagus. Biopsies confirm moderately differentiated squamous cell carcinoma. Which of the following is not needed to plan his treatment?

A) CT scan CAP

B) PET-CT scan

C) EUS

D) Staging laparoscopy

E) Discussion at MDM

Question 7

A 65 year old presents with a new onset dyspepsia not responding to PPI. You arrange an OGD. The report says a small growth is seen near OG junction and is biopsied. It is stated to be Siewert type II. What do you understand by this term?

A) It specifies degree of differentiation of the cancer cells, type II being moderately differentiated

B) It denotes location of the tumour as between 1 and 5cm above cardia

C) It is true junctional tumour within 1cm above and 2cm below the anatomical cardia

D) It suggests the tumour is not operable

E) The patient should have chemotherapy first

Question 8

A healthy 45 year old is found to have a submucosal gastric lump during OGD for dyspepsia. Biopsies show normal mucosa. CT scan and EUS are arranged and show it to be 6cm proximal gastric GIST along the fundus. Which of the following treatment options will be the best option for this patient?

A) Surveillance OGD every 2 years

B) OGD + EUS every year

C) Total gastrectomy + radical lymphnode dissection

D) Wedge resection the fundus ensuring tumour-free margins

E) Glivec (Imatinib) orally

Question 9

A 10-year-old child presents to A&E with history of foreign body ingestion. X-ray shows an object in oesophagus. Which of the following is the correct indication to take the patient to theatre to attempt endoscopic removal of the foreign body?

A) The child has airway compromise

B) He is unable to swallow saliva

C) A button battery is seen in the mid oesophagus

D) It is more than 24 hours since ingestion of the foreign body

E) All the above

Question 10

A 75-year-old female patient presents with acute onset upper abdominal pain. She has no known comorbidities. After adequate resuscitation and analgesia a CT scan is performed. It shows a perforated duodenal ulcer and the radiologist thinks it is probably sealed. The patient has moderate free fluid in the abdomen. Her WCC is 18.2. Her pulse is 110/minute. She has soft abdomen with some tenderness in RUQ and epigastrium. Which of the following treatment options would you choose in this case?

A) Conservative with IV fluids and antibiotics

B) Laparoscopic washouts + omental patch repair

C) Open washouts and omental patch repair

D) Duodenal stent + fasting

E) CT guided drainage of the free fluid should suffice

Question 11

A 42-year-old man presents with chest and abdominal pain. He gives history of retching and violent vomiting after a large meal. He is clammy and sweating. His pulse is 118/minute, BP 140/90 and respiratory rate of 24/minute. He has abdominal tenderness and surgical emphysema in the neck. Auscultation reveals reduced air entry on the left. You suspect Boerhaave syndrome. A CT scan confirms the diagnosis. Which 2 of the following statements are correct?

    A) Patient should have immediate resuscitation, IV fluids, oxygen, antibiotics, antifungal and PPI given

    B) An OGD should be undertaken at earliest opportunity to assess the perforation and insert NG tube under vision

    C) Meckler's triad is diagnostic and its absence rules out the condition

    D) Usually there is a single long oesophageal perforation in lower anterolateral oesophagus on left side

    E) Conservative treatment is norm

Question 12

A 39-year-old woman is referred by GP to your outpatient clinic with severe heartburn symptoms and would like to consider antireflux surgery. OGD shows a 4cm sliding hiatus hernia with volume reflux. You arrange pH studies and manometry. Manometry shows hypotensive lower oesophageal sphincter and ineffective lower oesophageal peristalsis. Demeester score is high at 24. Which of the following factors are not included when calculating Demeester score?

    A) Total reflux

    B) Upright reflux

    C) Symptom index

    D) Longest reflux

    E) Supine reflux

Question 13

A 71-year-old unwell woman presents with chest discomfort around 10pm to A&E. She gives history of a large late evening meal followed by retching. She is known to have a hiatus hernia. She vomits coffee ground fluid. Her pulse rate is 124/minute, BP 80/60 RR 26/minute and lactate of 3.4. CT scan shows 2/3rd stomach in chest and you are worried she has gastric volvulus and ischaemia. What is best next step in her management after initial resuscitation?

A) Insert NG tube on ward, keep fasting and arrange OGD next day

B) Take patient to theatre immediately for OGD + NG tube insertion and to proceed with surgery if needed

C) Ask radiologist to arrange a barium swallow examination to asses her hiatus hernia further

D) Laparoscope the patient straight away

E) IV fluids, antibiotics, Oxygen and PPI; reassure the patient

Question 14

Which of the following is not an indication for urgent OGD referral as per latest NICE guidelines?

A) Chronic GI bleeding

B) Iron deficiency anaemia

C) Progressive dysphagia

D) Epigastric mass

E) Obstructive jaundice

Question 15

A 49-year-old man is admitted with UGI bleed. His OGD shows a bleeding duodenal ulcer that is treated with endoscopic duel therapy successfully. The patient develops a rebleed after 48 hours. What will be your response?

A) Wait and watch; blood transfusion as required

B) Another OGD with repeat endoscopic therapy to stop bleeding

C) Surgery

D) Interventional radiology for selective embolisation

E) Tranexamic acid 1 gm stat and 8 hourly for 24 hours

Question 16

A young man accidently swallows a corrosive caustic alkaline liquid. Which of the following actions will you undertake urgently?

A) PPI, fasting and give TPN for nutrition

B) Bedside wide bore NG tube insertion and aspiration

C) OGD while protecting airway

D) Contact poison centre and administer antidote orally

E) Contrast swallow examination

Question 17

Which of the following doesn't contribute to acid reflux prevention?

A) A negative intra-abdominal pressure on short intra-abdominal oesophagus

B) A high pressure zone at lower end of the oesophagus (called lower oesophageal sphincter)

C) Natural obliquity of the oesophago-gastric angle

D) Pinch-cock effect of crural sling of diaphragm

E) Mucosal folds at the cardiac orifice

Question 18

A 65-year-old woman is found to have a small mid-oesophageal malignant-looking lesion on Barrett's surveillance OGD. Biopsy confirms this to be moderately differentiated adenocarcinoma. The staging on CT scan is T2N1M0. What is the next investigation you would like to do before offering treatment?

A) Diagnostic laparoscopy

B) USS liver

C) All-body bone scan

D) EUS

E) Bronchoscopy

Question 19

The above patient (as in question 18) has final staging as T2N0M0. Which of the following treatment options will be the best option?

    A) Endoscopic resection

    B) Radical chemo-radiotherapy

    C) Neoadjuvant chemotherapy as per CROSS protocol

    D) Ivor Lewis oesophagectomy

    E) Staging laparoscopy first

Extended Matching Question 20 – Oesophago-gastric Cancer Treatment

    a) Radical chemo-radiotherapy ☐

    b) Palliative chemotherapy ☐

    c) Neoadjuvant chemotherapy ☐

    d) Salvage oesophagectomy ☐

    e) Palliation only ☐

    f) Endoscopic mucosal resection ☐

    g) Stent insertion ☐

    h) Total gastrectomy ☐

    i) Ivor-Lewis oesophago-gastrectomy ☐

    j) Gastro-jejunostomy ☐

    k) Partial gastrectomy ☐

For each of the following descriptions, choose the single most likely option from the list above. Each option may be used once, more than once or not at all.

1) An 86-year-old cachexic patient with arthritis, DM II, COPD and cardiac stents presents with progressive dysphagia. She is unable to eat. Her investigations show a stenosing growth in lower oesophagus with staging T4N2M1.

2) A 66-year-old man has been diagnosed to have T3N1M0 adenocarcinoma of the oesophagus. His CPEX shows anaerobic threshold of 13.

3) A 73-year-old female patient has developed recent onset intermittent difficulty swallowing. Urgent OGD shows upper oesophageal growth. Biopsies confirm moderately differentiated squamous cell cancer. The staging is T2N1M0.

4) A 56-year-old fit man has proximal gastric (Siewert type 3) adenocarcinoma not extending on to the cardia. TNM stage T2N0M0. Staging laparoscopy shows no metastasis.

5) A 58-year-old patient with lower oesophageal adeno carcinoma has had neoadjuvant chemotherapy. Restaging investigations show stable disease with no progression.

6) A 74-year-old patient presents with residual squamous cancer on endoscopic biopsies after radical chemo-radiotherapy.

7) A 93-year-old presents with UGI bleeding and OGD shows a large ulcerated growth in body of stomach. Staging CT scan shows extensive disease with peritoneal metastasis.

8) A 78 year old on Barrett's surveillance program has developed an early Barrett's cancer with staging T1a.

9) An 87 year old who presents with fullness on meals and repeated vomiting is found to have antral cancer with gastric outlet obstruction. The patient is deemed not fit for major resectional surgery. He is keen to be able to eat and drink normally.

10) A 64-year-old patient presents with dyspepsia. OGD and staging investigations reveal an adenocarcinoma of lower oesophagus stage T3N1M1.

Question 21

Which of the following statements regarding UGI bleeding is correct?

A) Varices are the cause in over half the cases

B) Malignancy accounts for around 25% cases

C) Oesophagitis accounts for only 2% cases

D) Peptic ulcers are the most common cause of bleeding

E) Mallory–Weiss tear causes trivial bleeding and never presents as hematemesis

Question 22

Which of the factors mentioned below is not used in the Rockall scoring system to predict rebleeding or death risk in non-variceal UGI haemorrhage cases?

A) Age >90

B) Pulse >100

C) BP <100 mm Hg

D) Disseminated malignancy

E) Stigmata of recent bleeding

Question 23

A patient gets unwell 2 days post oesophagectomy with reduced oxygen saturation and sepsis. Which of the following is unlikely to be the complication responsible for these changes.

A) Pneumonia

B) Anastomotic leak

C) Anastomotic stricture

D) Gastric conduit necrosis

E) Broncho-pleural fistula

Question 24

The following are all true of gastric cancer except:

A) In the West, it affects distal and proximal stomach equally

B) Blood group A and H pylori are the risk factors

C) Previous gastric surgery is a risk factor

D) Microsatellite instability is implicated in the pathogenesis

E) High-fibre diet is protective

Question 25

You see a 74-year-old farmer in your clinic with a 4-week history of difficulty swallowing, loss of weight and appetite. An OGD shows a large submucosal lesion at the GOJ area. What of the following is not a prognostic indicator?

A) Size of the tumour

B) Site of the tumour in GI tract

C) Mitotic index

D) Bleeding surface

E) KIT and DOG positivity

Question 26

What is the most common presentation of a GIST?

A) Bleeding

B) Pain

C) Obstruction

D) Incidental

E) Weight loss

Question 27

A 37-year-old woman has refractory benign peptic ulcers despite high-dose PPI treatment over many months. You are concerned she has Zollinger Ellison syndrome. Which of the following is not a diagnostic test for a gastrinoma?

A) Gastrin level

B) Secretin stimulation test

C) C-peptide suppression test

D) Chromogranin A

E) CT – pancreatic protocol

F) EUS + Octreotide scan

Question 28

All are true about PET-CT except:

A) Patients need to fast 6 hours before the scan

B) It should be used in staging investigations of all cases of oesophageal cancer

C) It is not very informative and hence not used for gastric cancer staging

D) It uses orthovoltage X-rays and radioactive glucose

E) The cost is approximately £1,000 per patient

Question 29

A 36-year-old executive presents with persistent reflux symptoms. Omeprazole helps the symptoms but he hates to take medication. His OGD shows 4cm sliding hiatus hernia and grade I oesophagitis. The pH studies show Demeester score of 28. What is the best course of action?

A) Laparoscopic Nissen's fundoplication

B) Laparoscopic gastropexy

C) Open Nissen's fundoplication

D) Antireflux lifestyle, avoid late-evening large meals, regular PPI

E) LINX procedure

Question 30

A 49-year-old alcoholic presents with upper GI bleeding episodes. He is diagnosed to have portal hypertension and oesophageal varices. Which of the following is not an accepted method of treating varices?

A) Endoscopic banding

B) TIPSS

C) Terlipressin

D) Sengstaken tube

E) Transection and reanastomosis of oesophagogastric junction

Question 31

A patient with oesophagectomy developes chylothorax 3 days postoperatively. Which of the following statements is not correct about the condition?

    A) It is caused by damage to thoracic duct during the surgery

    B) It presents usually in first week after surgery especially when patient commences oral intake

    C) It should be treated by prompt return to theatre

    D) It causes malnutrition and immune suppression from loss of CD4+ white cells

    E) Patients benefit from enterally fed medium chain triglycerides

Question 32

A 48-year-old lady presents in the middle of night with sudden onset dysphagia. She has been unable to swallow solids and liquids for the last 24 hours. She gives history of gastric band insertion at the regional bariatric centre 8 months back and readjustment last week. Clinically she is stable. You suspect a tight gastric band. What will be your first step in her management?

    A) X-ray chest and abdomen

    B) Empty the balloon with a Huber needle

    C) Barium swallow examination

    D) CT scan with oral contrast

    E) Laparoscopy and gastric-band removal

Question 33

Which one of the following is not an indication for offering bariatric surgery?

    A) BMI over 40

    B) BMI over 35 with comorbidity that will benefit from weight loss

    C) BMI of 30–35 with inadequately controlled diabetes

    D) For Asian and other ethnicities with increased risk, the BMI limit is brought down by 5

    E) Patient has tried all appropriate non-surgical measures and failed to achieve or maintain adequate, clinically beneficial weight loss for at least 6 months

CHAPTER 13
HPB SURGERY

Answers on page 262–278

Mr Roland Fernandes
MBBS BSc FRCS
General and UGI Surgeon
East Kent Hospital University Foundation Trust

Question 1

A 76-year-old patient is admitted with painless jaundice, weight
loss and liver function tests of bilirubin 65, alkaline phosphatase
401, ALT 102 and albumin 32. What would be the most useful initial
investigation?

    A) Ultrasound abdomen

    B) CT CAP

    C) MRCP

    D) EUS

    E) ERCP

Question 2

A 67-year-old woman presents with vague abdominal discomfort and
liver function tests of bilirubin 56, alkaline phosphatase 305, ALT 201
and albumin 34. What would be the most useful initial investigation?

    A) Ultrasound abdomen

    B) CT CAP

    C) MRCP

    D) EUS

    E) ERCP

Question 3

A 76-year-old patient is admitted with upper abdominal discomfort, jaundice and liver function tests of bilirubin 65, alkaline phosphatase 401, ALT 102 and albumin 32. His ultrasound has revealed sludge within the gallbladder, a CBD of 12mm and no overt choledocholithiasis but the distal common bile duct could not be seen. What would be the next most useful initial investigation?

    A) Repeat ultrasound abdomen

    B) CT CAP

    C) MRCP

    D) EUS

    E) ERCP

Question 4

A 38-year-old woman who underwent a laparoscopic cholecystectomy 6 years ago presents with ongoing right upper quadrant pain and normal liver function tests. She has had an ultrasound that has revealed a common bile duct of 6mm. What would be the most appropriate investigation?

    A) Repeat ultrasound

    B) MRI liver

    C) OGD

    D) HIDA scan

    E) MRCP

Question 5

What does HIDA stand for?

    A) Hepatobiliary iminodiacetic acid scan

    B) Hydroxycarbamine induced delay assessment

    C) Hepatobiliary induced delay assessment

    D) Hydroxycarbamine iminodiacetic acid scan

    E) Hepatocholecystic indirect assessment

Question 6

Which of the following is an absolute contraindication to an HIDA scan?

- A) Pregnancy
- B) Breastfeeding
- C) Renal failure
- D) Previous HIDA scan within the last 12 months
- E) Hypersensitivity to hepatobiliary radioactive compound

Question 7

A 61-year-old woman presents with painless jaundice and a bilirubin of 201. Her CT and MRCP reveal a suspected ampullary tumour with liver metastases. Prior to her admission she had an active lifestyle and is keen for all treatment available. What do you think the recommendation would be following MDT discussion?

- A) ERCP with metal stent and brushings
- B) ERCP with plastic stent and brushings
- C) Whipple's operation
- D) Palliation
- E) PTC

Question 8

Which of the following has been proven to reduce the incidence of post ERCP pancreatitis?

- A) Pre-procedure diclofenac PR
- B) Pre-procedure diclofenac orally
- C) Pre-procedure gentamicin
- D) Post-procedure gentamicin
- E) Peri-procedure IV Buscopan

Question 9

What would be the ideal management of a patient presenting with acute right upper quadrant pain of 36-hour duration with known gallstones and normal blood results, who is on the waiting list for a laparoscopic cholecystectomy?

    A) Analgesia and acute laparoscopic cholecystectomy

    B) Analgesia, discharge and awaiting elective surgery

    C) Analgesia and repeat ultrasound

    D) MRCP to exclude choledocholithasis

    E) CT to exclude other pathology

Question 10

A 42-year-old woman presents with a 3-day history of acute epigastric pain. Blood tests show bil 17, alk phos 52, ALT 32, alb 34, wcc 12, CRP 52. An ultrasound has shown gallstones, thickened gallbladder wall and no biliary dilatation. What would be the next appropriate step?

    A) Antibiotics and laparoscopic cholecystectomy after 6 weeks

    B) Antibiotics with acute laparoscopic cholecystectomy

    C) Cholecystostomy

    D) ERCP

    E) Antibiotics and review in clinic

Question 11

A 92-year-old woman presents with a 3-day history of acute epigastric pain. Blood tests show bil 17, alk phos 52, ALT 32, alb 34, wcc 22, CRP 452. An ultrasound has shown a hugely dilated gallbladder, gallstones, thickened gallbladder wall and no biliary dilatation. She is frail and has multiple comorbidities but both the patient and her family are keen for "all to be done". What would be the next appropriate step?

    A) Antibiotics and laparoscopic cholecystectomy after 6 weeks

    B) Antibiotics with acute laparoscopic cholecystectomy

    C) Cholecystostomy

    D) ERCP

    E) Antibiotics and review in clinic

Question 12

A 55-year-old man presents septic with acute upper abdominal pain. He reports dark urine and pale stools. He is requiring inotropes on ITU as a consequence of his sepsis. An ultrasound has shown gallstones and biliary dilatation. An MRCP has shown a CBD of 9mm with choledocholiathiasis. What would you recommend?

A) Acute laparoscopic/open cholecystectomy + OTC + bile duct exploration

B) Open cholecystectomy

C) Cholecystostomy

D) ERCP

E) PTC

Question 13

The splenic notch is located on which border of the spleen?

A) Inferomedial

B) Inferolateral

C) Anteromedial

D) Anterolateral

E) Superolateral

Question 14

The splenic vein drains directly into the:

A) Portal vein

B) Superior mesenteric vein

C) Inferior mesenteric vein

D) Left gastric vein

E) Left gastroepiploic vein

Question 15

The following are all causes of splenomegaly except:

A) Portal vein thrombosis

B) Sickle cell

C) Hereditary spherocytosis

D) Schistosomiasis

E) ITP idiopathic thrombocytopenic purpura

Question 16

Which of the following is false with regard to hydatid cysts?

A) The organism usually responsible is echinococcus granulosus

B) They ostly occur in the right lobe of the liver

C) Gharbi's classification is used to describe their nature

D) Open surgery is contraindicated

E) The PAIR procedure refers to Puncture, Aspirate – if no bile – Inject (ethanol 95%), Reaspirate x 3 times

Question 17

According to the Csendes classification, how many types of Mirrizi syndrome are there?

A) 1

B) 2

C) 3

D) 4

E) 5

Question 18

With regard to choledochal cysts, which of the following statements is false?

A) Usually presents in middle age

B) There is a 12% risk of adenocarcinoma

C) Liver resection is sometimes required

D) The Todani classification describes 5 types

E) Caroli Disease (Type V) describes intrahepatic cystic disease

Question 19

What is the approximate risk of bile duct injury in a laparoscopic cholecystectomy?

A) 1/10

B) 1/50

C) 1/100

D) 1/200

E) 1/500

Question 20

Which of the following is a common classification system used in bile-duct injuries?

    A) Strasberg
    B) Csendes
    C) Bismuth
    D) Todani
    E) Bismuth-Corlette

Question 21

Klatsin cholangiocarcinoma refers to which bile-duct malignancy?

    A) Bile-duct confluence
    B) Intrahepatic
    C) Distal bile duct
    D) Refers to the histology rather than site of malignancy
    E) None of the above

Question 22

Which of the following arteries arise from the superior mesenteric artery?

    A) Gastroduodenal artery
    B) Left gastroepiploic artery
    C) Splenic artery
    D) Superior pancreaticoduodenal artery
    E) Inferior pancreaticoduodenal artery

Question 23

Which of the following is not part of the Atlanta classification for the diagnosis of pancreatitis?

    A) Amylase 3 times the upper limit of normal
    B) CRP 3 times the upper limit of normal
    C) Epigastric pain
    D) Lipase 3 times the upper limit of normal
    E) Characteristic imaging findings on CT/MRI

Question 24

Which of the following is not part of the Glasgow Imrie criteria?

A) PaO2 <8kPa

B) Wcc >11mmol/L

C) LDH >600iU/L

D) Urea >16mmol/L

E) Glucose >10mmol/L

Question 25

Which of the following has been shown to improve outcomes in pancreatitis?

A) Early enteral feeding

B) Antibiotics

C) TPN

D) Laparoscopic cholecystectomy during index admission if gallstone aetiology

E) Consultant review within 12 hours of admission

Question 26

Which of the following is a risk factor for pancreatic cancer?

A) Chronic pancreatitis

B) Lynch syndrome

C) MEN 1

D) FAP

E) All of the above

Question 27

What is the most common pancreatic cancer pathology?

A) Serous cystadenoma

B) IPMN – intraductal papillary neoplasm

C) Pancreatic endocrine tumour

D) Ductal adenocarcinoma

E) Mucinous cystadenocarcinoma

Question 28

How many anastomoses are there in a Whipple's pancreaticoduodenectomy?

    A) 1

    B) 2

    C) 3

    D) 4

    E) 5

Question 29

How many anastomoses are there in a pylorus preserving pancreaticoduodenectomy?

    A) 1

    B) 2

    C) 3

    D) 4

    E) 5

Question 30

Which of these pancreatic cystic tumours has the least malignant potential?

    A) Multiple branch IPMN

    B) Mucinous cystadenoma/carcinoma (MCN)

    C) Serous cystadenoma SCN

    D) Main duct IPMN

    E) Mixed variant

Question 31

What is the name of the classification system commonly used for IPMNs and MCNs?

    A) Balthazer

    B) Taneka

    C) Manoka

    D) Olivia Rose Burke

    E) Blumgart

Question 32

The majority of pancreatic neuroendocrine tumours are:

A) Non functional

B) Gastrinomas

C) Insulinomas

D) Carcinoids

E) Metastases

Question 33

Which of the following is inconsistent with a diagnosis of Zollinger Ellison Syndrome?

A) Recurrent peptic ulceration despite proton pump inhibitor therapy

B) Gastrin levels >1,000 with gastric pH <2.5

C) Ulcers in duodenum, stomach and atypical sites

D) Fall in gastrin levels following exogenous secretin

E) Endoscopic ultrasound findings consistent with a gastrinoma

Question 34

Which of the following is true with regard to glucagonomas?

A) Rise from the beta cells of the pancreas

B) 90% are benign

C) Weight gain is a feature

D) Somatostatin analogues and surgical resection are the mainstay of treatment

E) Glucagon levels <1,000 are a feature

Question 35

Which Couinaud segments form the right lobe of the liver?

A) 4, 5, 6 and 7

B) 1, 4, 5, 6 and 7

C) 2, 3 and 4

D) 5, 6, 7 and 8

E) 1, 2, 3, 4, 5 and 6

Question 36

Which Couinaud segments lie to the right of Cantlie's line?

A) 5, 6, 7 and 8

B) 1, 5, 6, 7 and 8

C) 1, 2, 3 and 4

D) 5, 6 and 7

E) 2, 3 and 4

Question 37

Which of the following is not a risk factor for the development of HCC?

A) Aflatoxins

B) Hepatitis C

C) Obesity

D) Haemochromatosis

E) Echinococcus granulosus

Question 38

Which of the following is not a pathological characteristic of HCC?

A) Lack of a distinct fibrous capsule

B) Presence of immunomarker heatshock protein 70

C) Arterial neoangiogenesis

D) Presence of immunomarker glutamine synthetase (G3)

E) Presence of immunomarker glypican 3 (GPC3)

Question 39

Which of these is not a feature you would expect to see on a triple phase CT on a patient with a HCC?

A) Washout of nodule on venous phase

B) Hyper-arterialisation on arterial phase

C) Satellite lesions

D) Bright dot sign

E) Rim enhancement on delayed post-contrast images

Question 40

The following are all licensed treatments for HCC, except:

A) TACE – trans arterial chemoembolisation

B) SIRT – selective internal radiotherapy

C) Oral sorafenib

D) Radiofrequency ablation

E) Liver resection

Question 41

Assuming the patient is fit, what is the only absolute contraindication to liver resection for a colorectal liver metastases?

A) Locoregional recurrence

B) Inadequate future liver remnant

C) Bone metastases

D) Non-treatable primary

E) Peritoneal disease

Question 42

In the Pringle manoeuver, which structure or structures are occluded?

A) Hepatic artery

B) Hepatic artery and portal vein

C) Portal vein and common bile duct

D) Portal vein

E) Hepatic artery, portal vein and common bile duct

Question 43

Which of the following is a cause for post-sinusoidal portal hypertension?

A) Portal vein thrombosis

B) Schistosomiasis

C) Budd–Chiari syndrome

D) Primary biliary cirrhosis

E) Haemochromatosis

Question 44

Which of the following is not a component of the Child–Pugh classification of cirrhosis?

  A) Prothrombin time
  B) Creatinine
  C) Bilirubin
  D) Albumin
  E) Hepatic encephalopathy

Extended Matching Question 45

  a) Acute infection ☐
  b) Haemangioma ☐
  c) Susceptible to infection ☐
  d) Chronic infection ☐
  e) Focal nodular hyperplasia ☐
  f) Immune following vaccination ☐
  g) Liver abscess ☐
  h) Immune following natural infection ☐
  i) HCC ☐
  j) Hepatic adenoma ☐

Match the following hepatitis serology results to the corresponding diagnosis:

1)

Hepatitis B surface antigen (HbsAg)	negative
Hepatitis B surface antibody (Anti-HBs)	negative
Hepatitis B core antibody (Anti-HBc)	negative
IgM antibody to hepatitis B core antigen (IgM anti-HBc)	negative

2)

Hepatitis B surface antigen (HbsAg)	positive
Hepatitis B surface antibody (Anti-HBs)	negative
Hepatitis B core antibody (Anti-HBc)	positive
IgM antibody to hepatitis B core antigen (IgM anti-HBc)	negative

3)

Hepatitis B surface antigen (HbsAg)	positive
Hepatitis B surface antibody (Anti-HBs)	negative
Hepatitis B core antibody (Anti-HBc)	positive
IgM antibody to hepatitis B core antigen (IgM anti-HBc)	positive

4)

Hepatitis B surface antigen (HbsAg)	negative
Hepatitis B surface antibody (Anti-HBs)	positive
Hepatitis B core antibody (Anti-HBc)	negative
IgM antibody to hepatitis B core antigen (IgM anti-HBc)	negative

5)

Hepatitis B surface antigen (HbsAg)	negative
Hepatitis B surface antibody (Anti-HBs)	positive
Hepatitis B core antibody (Anti-HBc)	positive
IgM antibody to hepatitis B core antigen (IgM anti-HBc)	negative

Match the following description to the most likely corresponding diagnosis

6) 66-year-old male with alcoholic-related cirrhosis

7) 50-year-old male with worsening RUQ pain and deranged LFTS over the last week

8) 33-year-old woman with an incidental lesion picked up on a MRI scan with a central scar

9) 31-year-old woman on the oral contraceptive pill with a hyper enhancing liver nodule

CHAPTER 14
COLORECTAL SURGERY

Answers on page 279–288

Mr Gandrasupalli Harinath
MB BS; MS, MPhil, FRCS (Gen)
Consultant General and Colorectal Surgeon
William Harvey Hospital, Ashford

COLOPROCTOLOGY QUESTIONS

Question 1

A 68-year-old male patient presents to A&E with massive dark PR bleeding. He was tachycardic, hypotensive and pale. The following initial management is appropriate except:

A) Crystalloid administration

B) Cross match of blood

C) Bowel preparation followed by urgent colonoscopy

D) Urgent intravenous administration of tranexamic acid

E) Urgent CT angiogram and interventional radiology consultation

Question 2

70-year-old female with a history of smoking presents with persisting anal ulceration with pain for 3 months. The following is correct except:

A) Botox treatment is not preferred initial management option

B) Discontinue if patient is on drugs such as nicorandil

C) Urgent lateral sphincterotomy is the primary surgical option

D) Secondary causes of ulceration need to be excluded by biopsy

E) Manual anal dilatation results in significant faecal incontinence

Question 3

The following management is appropriate in acute pouchitis patients except:

    A) Pouch biopsy is useful

    B) A course of oral metronidazole is initial management of choice

    C) No correlation with eventual pouch failure

    D) Predicts likely future poucitis

    E) VSL# 3 is indicated

Question 4

A 75-year-old gentleman had low anterior resection with defunctioning loop ileostomy 5 days ago. He is tachycardic with pyrexia. The following statements are correct except:

    A) Urgent CT scan with rectal contrast to rule out anastomotic leak is essential

    B) Normal WCC and CRP do not rule out anastomotic leak

    C) Conservative management on the assumption that this is ileus or atelectasis is appropriate

    D) Laparoscopic approach is reasonable to deal with the anastomotic leak

    E) If patient has leaked from anastomosis, it is possible to preserve the anastomosis in select cases

Question 5

In the treatment of anal cancer, which of the following statements is true?

    A) There is no significant difference in the outcomes following radiotherapy versus combined chemo-radiotherapy

    B) Rectus abdominis flap is a useful approach to close the perineal defect following salvage surgical resection

    C) Incidence of primary treatment failure with combined chemo-radiotherapy is up to 40%

    D) Posterior vaginal wall involvement on MRI scan is a contraindication for salvage AP resection

    E) Inguinal lymph node involvement is considered as contraindication for initial chemo-radiotherapy

Question 6

A 79-year-old vasculopath presents with sudden severe abdominal pain in the lower abdomen on the left side. He also passed a large amount of dark rectal bleed. His white cell counts are 26, CRP 400. Blood gases revealed acidosis with raised lactate at 4.9. The next most appropriate management in this patient is:

A) Initial resuscitation followed by urgent CT scan abdomen and pelvis

B) Urgent laparotomy to assess bowel

C) Colonoscopic assessment of the left colon to rule out ischaemic colitis

D) Urgent interventional radiology consultation to angio-embolise to stop bleeding

E) Conservative management with therapeutic dose clexane and haematology opinion

Question 7

In the management of a patient with familial adenomatous polyposis, which of the following is correct?

A) Colonoscopic screening must start by the age of 40

B) Abdominal desmoids do not impair formation of ileal pouch

C) Total colectomy and formation of ileal pouch protects the patient against future gastrointestinal polyps

D) FAP pouches are less likely to develop pouchitis than colitic pouches

E) Some FAP patients never develop small bowel polyps

Question 8

In the treatment of recurrent rectal cancer, which of the following is false?

A) FD-PET scan is useful prior to planning surgical resection

B) Involvement of S3 and anterior sacral foramen is a contraindication for radical resection

C) Bone scan is essential prior to embarking radical resection

D) Radical resection is a multidisciplinary approach involving orthopaedic, neuro and plastic surgeons.

E) Involvement of bladder base is not a contraindication

Question 9

A 40-year-old male presents with primary fissure in ano with 3 months of symptoms. Which of the following is correct with regards to the GTN treatment?

A) Response rates with GTN treatment are comparable to those of lateral internal sphincterotomy

B) Compliance rate is 90%

C) Dose escalation studies confirm improvement in response rates

D) Long-term response rates are poor

E) GTN acts through muscuranic receptors

Question 10

A 50-year-old multiparous woman has been diagnosed with a chronic fissure in ano. The following statements are applicable in the management except:

A) Non-resolution of fissure in ano is an indication for examination and anaesthetic with biopsy if indicated

B) Excision of fissure with advancement flap is the initial treatment of choice in this patient

C) Dose escalation with GTN has been shown to improve the outcomes

D) Lateral sphincterotomy carries risk of incontinence in the long term

E) Multiple fissures could suggest secondary aetiology

Question 11

In the case of a 75-year-old lady with a 4-year history of significant incontinence, the following are reasonable initial management options except:

A) Endo-anal assessment and anal manometry

B) Conservative treatment trial with diet and immodium

C) Flexible sigmoidoscopy to exclude any left colonic lesion

D) Tertiary referral to consider sphincter repair or dynamic graciloplasty

E) Counsel for colostomy: this is the last option

Question 12

In the chemo-prevention of colorectal cancers, the following are correct except:

A) Aspirin may prevent colorectal polyp formation

B) Sulindac has been shown to reduce adenomatous polyp formation in the colon

C) Cyclooxygenase 2 pathway is the chief pathway to prevent cancers and high risk adenomas

D) COX 1 is expressed in 90% of colorectal cancers

E) Ingestion of multivitamin pills does not reduce overall prevalence of colorectal polyps

Question 13

A 40-year-old female had a right hemicolectomy for a right colon cancer. HNPCC was suspected. The following statements are true of the management of this patient except:

A) Referral to gynaecologist to consider prophylactic hysterectomy

B) MSI testing is indicated

C) Signet ring of cancer is more likely on histological examination

D) Ophthalmology referral is indicated to check for CHRPE

E) HNPCC associated colonic cancers have better survival compared to sporadic colon cancers

Question 14

A 40-year-old male presents with family history of bowel cancers with 2 first-degree relatives under 40 and one second-degree relative above 50 with bowel cancer. He is asymptomatic. Which of the following is most appropriate?

A) Baseline colonoscopy

B) Faecal immunochemical test

C) Regular aspirin for long-term management

D) Rigid sigmoidoscopy

E) Regular vitamin E intake

Question 15

A 25-year-old young lady has been referred for consideration of ileo-anal pouch following total colectomy for colitis 6 months ago. The following are relevant in the management except:

A) Establishing accurate histological diagnosis to ensure there was no Crohn's or indeterminate colitis

B) Thorough counselling with stoma nurses and education through pouch forums

C) Explain to patient that pouch surgery is risky and reject surgery

D) Ask patient to complete family before considering pouch surgery

E) Pouch surgery may be carried out laparoscopically

Question 16

Select the true statement with regards to familial adenomatous polyposis:

A) 50% of cases develop desmoid tumours

B) Fundoscopic examination for congenital hypertrophic retinal pigment epithelium (CHRPE) is useful prior to genetic testing

C) Rectal cancer risk following total colectomy and ileorectal anastomosis can be eradicated by NSAIDs

D) Small-bowel enteroscopy may be necessary in select cases

E) Total colonoscopy and transvaginal US should be performed early on as a part of screening strategy

Question 17

The following surgical principles are widely practised in the surgical treatment of rectal cancer except:

A) Routine high tie of the IMA pedicle

B) Routine washing of the residual rectum

C) All rectal cancers will need 5cm of distal clearance

D) Anastomotic leaks can be prevented by routine ileostomy

E) Laparoscopic TME surgery carries an increased risk of local and port site recurrence

Question 18

The following statements are true concerning gastrointestinal stromal tumours (GIST) except:

A) With appropriate strategy GIST can be prevented

B) Patients with neurofibromatosis type 1 are at increased risk of GIST

C) Imatinib can be used in neo-adjuvant and adjuvant settings

D) Surgery is the standard treatment of choice

E) Often biopsy is required to make a diagnosis

Question 19

Concerning the follow-up of colorectal cancer patients, which of the following is false?

A) Intense follow-up is inappropriate in all cases

B) Regular follow-up has been shown to increase detection of resectable hepatic metastatic disease

C) Colonoscopic surveillance is appropriate

D) Clinical examination is not enough to establish early local recurrence following rectal cancer excision

E) Routine CEA assessment is indicated during follow-up period.

Question 20

Concerning screening of colorectal cancers, which of the following statements is false?

A) Screening has been shown to reduce mortality

B) Screening programme is more likely to detect early cancers

C) The screening programme is cost effective

D) Faecal immunochemical test is superior to faecal occult blood test

E) Flexible sigmoidoscopy is optimum screening test in families with HNPCC

Question 21

HNPCC is associated with the following, except:

A) Adenomatous polyps in the colon

B) Right-sided tumours are more common

C) Retinal pigment abnormalities

D) Extracolonic tumours such as endometrial and ovarian cancers

E) Tumours have marked lymphocytic infiltration

Question 22

Which of the following is true concerning anal intra-epithelial neoplasia?

A) Natural history of majority of AIN is inevitable development of anal cancer

B) AIN III detected on histology of the haemorrhoidal tissue is treated with radical combined chemo-radiotherapy

C) Human papilloma virus strain 2 is more likely to be associated with AIN III than other cutaneous papillomata

D) Ulcerated type of AIN III is treated primarily with topical 5-FU

E) Lesions such as VIN, VAIN and CIN pathologies could co-exist

Question 23

A 55-year-old lady presented with a 3-year history of constipation. She has opened her bowels once in 2 weeks. She has no daily urge. Which of the following is false?

A) Defecating proctogram and colon transit studies are essential for assessment

B) 5 HT4 agonist is the treatment of choice if dietary measures and laxatives fail

C) Initial management of choice is a high-fibre diet and biofeedback

D) Subtotal colectomy has good results for functional disease

E) Rectocele and or intussusception could be contributing to symptoms

Question 24

A 75-year-old man undergoes open AAA repair. On the second post-operative day, he complains of abdominal pain with bloody diarrhoea. His WCC is raised at 14 with raised CRP of 125. The following is appropriate management except:

A) Urgent CT scan abdomen

B) Consider anticoagulating the patient

C) Intravenous tranexamic acid to minimise PR blood loss

D) Flexible sigmoidoscopic assessment of the left colon

E) Emergency laparotomy may be necessary if colon was found to be irreversibly ischaemic

Question 25

A 25-year-old man undergoes proctectomy and ileo-anal pouch for ulcerative colitis. On the fifth post-operative day, he becomes septic. Which of the following statement is false concerning this clinical management?

A) A CT scan of the pelvis is indicated to exclude pouch-related sepsis

B) Temporary ileostomy is a surgical option if the pouch has leaked

C) Urgent pouch excision is indicated early in cases with pouch ischaemia

D) A defunctioning loop ileostomy would have prevented leak

E) Early pouch leak predicts subsequent development of pouchitis and subsequent pouch excision

Question 26

Concerning the gastrointestinal lymphomas, the following statements are true except:

A) B cell lymphomas are most common in the GI tract

B) T cell lymphomas are associated with malabsorption enteropathy

C) Gastric lymphomas are not associated with MEN-1 syndrome

D) MALT-omas are associated with H. pylori in 70–80% of cases

E) Imatinib is highly effective in the treatment of gastric lymphomas

Question 27

A 45-year-old male presented with central and lower abdominal pain of 3 months. An initial ultrasound scan and subsequent CT scan abdomen have confirmed 9cm intra-abdominal lump. This was closely associated with small bowel. The following are appropriate in the management of the patient except:

A) CT-guided biopsy is appropriate for confirming diagnosis

B) If confirmed as leiomyosarcoma then surgical resection is the primary modality of treatment

C) Selective tyrosine kinase inhibitor such as Glivec is the initial management of choice if GIST is confirmed on biopsy

D) Surgery is reserved for persisting GIST lumps; this may help to reduce the extent of resection

E) Gastrointestinal stromal tumours are more common in stomach than small bowel

Extended Matching Question 28

1) Haemorrhoids   ☐
2) Rectal prolapse   ☐
3) Fissure in ano   ☐
4) Fistula in ano   ☐
5) Proctalgia fugax   ☐
6) Crohn's disease perineum   ☐
7) Perianal skin tag   ☐
8) Pilonidal sinus   ☐
9) Solitary rectal ulcer syndrome   ☐
10) Rectocele   ☐

A) 40-year-old male with type 2 DM presents with intermittent anal pain with discomfort and blood stained discharge.

B) An 80-year-old multiparous lady presents with recurrent PR bleeding with protruded mass per anum.

C) 50-year-old lady presents with anal pain with PR bleeding of 2 month's duration. Pain is intense with throbbing following act of defecation.

D) 55-year-old lady with constipation of 2 years duration. There is daily urge but cannot evacuate, leading to digitation often. There is occasional PR bleeding on wiping.

E) 25-year-old young lady presents with perianal lump, no pain. No PR bleeding.

F) 45-year-old male with history of smoking presents with lump and discharge from the natal cleft. He has a few courses of antibiotics from his GP.

G) 20-year-old young lady with ileo-caecal Crohn's disease presents with perianal discomfort but minimal bleeding and discomfort. Occasional mucus and pus was also noted.

H) 55-year-old male lorry driver presents with intermittent PR bleeding for 3 years with some constipation. Bright bleeding after defecation. No other symptoms.

I) 50-year-old lady with anal pain of 3 years, intermittently. This is throbbing in nature. No associated symptoms such as PR bleeding. There is occasional pain even during night times with radiation. Anal spasms lasts for days on some occasions.

J) 50-year-old healthy female with chronic constipation with difficulty in evacuation also has tenesmus. She has 3/12 history of fresh PR bleeding with mucus on straining. History of digitation is also present.

Extended Matching Question 29

1) Irritable bowel syndrome ☐
2) Acute severe ulcerative colitis ☐
3) Obstructive defecation syndrome ☐
4) Faecal incontinence ☐
5) Complicated diverticular disease ☐

A) 38-year-old lady presents with intermittent diarrhoea with bloating in the abdomen. No PR bleeding symptoms reported. She also reports urgency and upper GI reflux. She notices some milk intolerance. No red flag symptoms.

B) 60-year-old lady with chronic constipation of 6 years duration. She opens bowels once in 2–3 weeks. There has been history of straining to evacuate unsuccessfully. On some occasions, she digitates to evacuate. She reports generalised bloating with lethargy.

C) 80-year-old elderly lady presents with 5 year history of incontinence. No previous surgery on anus. She had 3 normal deliveries. No difficult deliveries reported. Not diabetic. Not on any medications apart from some antihypertensives. Her Wexner incontinence score is 15.

D) 55-year-old male presents with acute abdominal pain in the left iliac fossa with tachycardia. Tenderness with some guarding noted locally. Not passed any blood PR; however, has been constipated for last 3 days.

E) 24-year-old female presents with acute abdominal pain with bloody diarrhoea up to 10 times a day. There was associated mucus and lethargy. WCC raised at 18 with CRP of 200.

Extended Matching Question 30

A) Anastomotic leak ☐

B) Paralytic ileus ☐

C) Atelectasis ☐

D) Pelvic collection ☐

E) Post-operative pneumonia ☐

1) A 75-year-old man undergoes laparoscopic converted to open low anterior resection with defunctioning loop ileostomy. On the 2nd post-operative day, he was tachycardic with temperature of 38 degrees. Abdominal examination showed mild distention, but non tender. There was no vomiting. NG aspirates are 50 mls of gastric juice. Temperature was 37.5. WCC risen to 14 with a CRP of 150. Lactate was 1.2. There was reduced air entry on both bases.

2) A 60-year-old male undergoes open extended right hemicolectomy for large splenic flexure carcinoma with an excision of cuff of greater curvature of stomach. There has been poor post-operative progress until 5th post day; there was large vomit of 1.5 litres of small bowel content. White cells raised at 12. Mild alkalosis with normal lactate noted on the blood gas analysis. There was temperature of 38 noted on one occasion. Respiratory examination showed some poor air entry in the bases. Abdominal examination revealed distention. Very few high pitched bowel sounds heard.

3) A 68-year-old male undergoes laparoscopic low anterior resection. Did not open bowels or pass flatus on 5th post-operative day. Patient was tachycardic, with white cell of 18. CRP raised to 250. Abdominal examination revealed distention with guarding. Lactate raised to 2.8.

4) A 78-year-old male with known COPD underwent right hemicolectomy through a transverse incision in the right side of the abdomen for cancer of the caecum. On the 3rd post-operative day, patient was tachypnoeic with HR 110, WCC raised to 18. Lactate was 1.2. Alkalotic. Hypoxia was noted. Chest examination revealed bronchial breathing in the right base with crackles in the left chest; there were also rhonchi.

5) A 65-year-old male chronic smoker with type II DM underwent high anterior resection for complicated diverticular disease with a stricture. On the 5th post-operative day, the patient was ill. He was tachycardic with diffuse lower abdominal tenderness but not peritonitic. WCC were raised at 16.5, CRP 200. Lactate was 1.8. Urine output was good; few bowel sounds heard.

Extended Matching Question 31

1) Capsule endoscopy ☐
2) Colonoscopy ☐
3) Flexible sigmoidoscopy ☐
4) FIT ☐
5) Rigid sigmoidoscopy ☐
6) Small-bowel enteroscopy ☐
7) Mesenteric angiogram ☐
8) CT angiogram ☐
9) NM colon transit studies ☐
10) PET scan ☐

A) A 42-year-old male with fresh PR bleeding of 3 months duration. This is associated with perianal irritation symptoms. No family history of bowel cancers or inflammatory bowel disease. No alteration of bowel was reported.

B) 60-year-old healthy male attends his GP with concern of bowel cancer in the family. He is asymptomatic. No other risk factors.

C) 68-year-old female with alteration of bowels with dark PR bleeding. Her grandmother died of bowel cancer at the age of 60. No first-degree relatives with bowel cancer. No weight loss reported.

D) 64-year-old lady had upper GI endoscopy and colonoscopy to investigate for iron deficiency anaemia. Both investigations were normal. Coeliac screen was negative, as was the duodenal biopsy. What is the next best investigation?

E) A 45-year-old lady had small-bowel MRI scan due to abdominal pain. This showed possible lesion 2cm in size in the mid small bowel. No history of long-term analgesic use. No Crohn's disease in the family. No loss of weight. No polyps in the family.

F) 20-year-old male presents with fresh PR bleeding of 2 months' duration. History of constipation was noted. No other symptoms noted. No family history of polyps or bowel cancer.

G) A 58-year-old lady presents with 5-year history of constipation. Opens bowels once in 2 to 3 weeks. There is associated straining and digitation. No sinister symptoms reported.

H) A 67-year-old male with confirmed rectal cancer has 2 liver lesions. Both lesions are in the right lobe. CT chest showed some indeterminate lesions in the left lung base. What is the best investigation to understand if there is any extra-hepatic disease?

I) 75-year-old male underwent endovascular stent for leaking abdominal aortic aneurysm 3 days ago. He is still critical with new onset acidosis with a lactate level of 3. White cells were 25. CRP = 400.

J) 59-year-old male with a history of smoking presents with massive dark PR bleeding. His upper GI endoscopy showed no significant abnormality. HB was 70 gms. Lactate 2.0. Mild alkalosis noted. What is the next best investigation?

CHAPTER 15
VASCULAR SURGERY

Answers on page 288–291

Mr Dean Godfrey
BM, PG Cert M Ed, MD(Res), FRCSEd (Gen-Vasc)
Consultant Vascular Surgeon, Dorset & Wiltshire Vascular Network

SINGLE BEST ANSWER

Question 1

Which branch of the abdominal aorta is most commonly affected by acute thromboembolic occlusion?

- A) Coeliac artery
- B) Superior Mesenteric artery
- C) Inferior Mesenteric artery
- D) Right renal artery
- E) Left renal artery

Question 2

Which of the following may be safely observed?

- A) Splenic artery aneurysm <20mm
- B) Asymptomatic mesenteric aneurysm in a woman of child-bearing age
- C) Hepatic artery aneurysm >25mm
- D) Abdominal aortic aneurysm 55mm
- E) Symptomatic aneurysm of the gastroduodenal artery >15mm

Question 3

Which of the following are considered first-line treatment in the management of great saphenous incompetence (with skin changes) in an otherwise-fit patient without confounding factors?

A) Foam sclerotherapy

B) Compression hosiery

C) Endovenous ablation

D) High tie and strip

E) Multiple avulsions

Question 4

A 34-year-old female on the combined oral contraceptive pill presents with acute left lower limb swelling, discolouration, pain without compromised viability. She is referred for a duplex and then a CT that confirms a focal common and iliac vein thrombosis with multiple pulmonary emboli. Which of the following would not be considered as management strategies at present?

A) IVC filter

B) Unfractionated heparin

C) Therapeutic low molecular weight heparin

D) Pharmaco-mechanical catheter directed thrombolysis

E) Palma procedure

Question 5

A patient presents with acute upper limb ischaemia (dominant) in the presence of a new onset of atrial fibrillation. She has a viable limb with diminished sensation and impaired motor function. The most appropriate management would be:

A) Therapeutic low molecular weight heparin

B) Unfractionated heparin

C) Compartment pressure assessment

D) Vascular imaging

E) Embolectomy

F) Fasciotomy

Question 6

A 78-year-old male with angina and lifestyle-limiting airways disease who underwent a femoro-distal bypass 3 years ago using autologous vein presents with recurrent sudden onset rest pain. A CT peripheral angiogram demonstrates a focal bypass graft occlusion with preserved inflow and outflow. The most appropriate management would be:

A) Unfractionated heparin

B) Systemic thrombolysis

C) Thromboembolectomy and vein patch plasty

D) Jump graft using short saphenous vein from ipsilateral limb

E) Catheter directed thrombolysis +/- proceed

F) Major limb amputation

Question 7

A male motorcyclist is admitted as a trauma with bilateral knee dislocations. Foot pulses were palpable on scene but are now only identified on one leg only. What is the likely cause for loss of pulses?

A) Compartment syndrome

B) Undiagnosed tibial/fibular fracture

C) Undiagnosed tibial plateau fracture

D) Buerger's disease

E) Intimal injury of popliteal artery

F) Fat embolism

Question 8

A patient presents with abdominal pain having undergone an elective endovascular aneurysm repair (EVAR) 12 months ago. A CT is performed which demonstrates a growth in aneurysm sac, without sign of rupture or secondary signs of infection or inflammation, with contrast flowing into the sac from the IMA and sacroiliac arteries. What endoleak type is this?

A) Type Ia

B) Type Ib

C) Type II

D) Type III

E) Type IV

F) Type V

Question 9

A 24-year-old male mechanic presents with acute limb swelling and discolouration to his dominant upper limb. There is no history of trauma and he is otherwise fit and well. Pulses are difficult to palpate owing to swelling but Doppler demonstrate triphasic signals in his radial and ulnar arteries. He has some venous dilatation across the deltoid region on examination but no other gross findings. The most likely diagnosis is:

    A) Neurogenic thoracic outlet syndrome

    B) Arterial thoracic outlet syndrome

    C) Paget–Schroetter syndrome

    D) Cervical rib

    E) Sympathetic dysregulation

Question 10

A patient who has recently been established on haemodialysis with a new brachio-basilic transposition fistula presents with finger-tip necrosis. The underlying patholophysiology is:

    A) Steal syndrome

    B) Small vessel disease

    C) Smoking

    D) Thromboangitis obliterans

    E) Microemboli

Question 11

Which of the following would gain most benefit from carotid endarterectomy in regards to future stroke risk reduction, assuming lateralising hemispherical symptomology within last two weeks?

    A) 55-year-old male with 100% occlusion of ICA

    B) 77-year-old male with 40% stenosis of ICA

    C) 64-year-old female with 50% stenosis of CCA

    D) 70-year-old male with 70% stenosis of ICA

    E) 89-year-old female with 75% stenosis of ICA

Question 12

A patient is taken to theatre for drainage of an active diabetic foot infection without vascular compromise. What is the most likely organism to be cultured?

    A) Staphylococcus

    B) Pseudomonas

    C) Proteus

    D) Streptococcus

    E) Escherichia coli

    F) Klebsiella

Question 13

A patient with a history of stable claudication at 100 metres presents via ED with an acute deterioration and now complains of rest pain and a sunset foot. The most likely cause of deterioration is:

    A) Deep vein thrombosis

    B) May–Thurner syndrome

    C) In-situ thrombosis

    D) Distal arterial emboli

    E) Autonomic dysregulation

Question 14

A patient with an arteriovenous fistula presents via ED with a bleed from a recent dialysis 'needling' site. There is a small patch of necrosis with surrounding erythema and a large pulsatile mass with palpable thrill below. The patient's observations are normal. You are asked for advice on management as the dialysis team who manage fistulae at your site "have a gap in their rota tonight". What is your advice?

    A) Check bloods and discharge if normal

    B) Discharge with antibiotics

    C) Discharge and liaise with dialysis team in the morning

    D) Admit for antibiotics

    E) Apply a tourniquet and transfer to ED clinical decision unit

EXTENDED MATCHING

Question 15

1) Ankle brachial pressure index (ABPI) ☐
2) Arterial duplex (non-dynamic) ☐
3) CT angiogram (abdominal aorta – femoral bifurcation) ☐
4) Downstream angiogram ☐
5) Pharmaco-mechanical catheter directed thrombolysis ☐
6) Lymphscintography ☐
7) Reflux venous duplex lower limb ☐
8) CT abdomen/pelvis ☐
9) HbA1c ☐
10) MR angiogram (peripheral) ☐

In the following scenarios, which of the options would be the most appropriate initial investigation/management?

A) 65-year-old male attends outpatient with non-lifestyle limiting intermittent claudication

B) 54-year-old female with a family history of DVT presents with phlegmasia

C) 12-year-old male presents with progressive leg swelling from birth

D) 62-year-old male diabetic patient with buttock pain and impotence

E) 24-year-old male soldier with bilateral calf claudication with ABPI drop post-exercise

F) 48-year-old female presents with peripheral neuropathy and ABPI >1.2

Question 16

Choose the preferred conduit in the following situations:

1) Autologous superficial vein – leg ☐
2) Prosthetic graft ☐
3) Silver impregnated graft ☐
4) Deep femoral vein ☐
5) Panel graft using bovine pericardial patch ☐

6) Javid shunt ☐

7) Radial artery ☐

8) Autologous vein – arm ☐

9) None ☐

10) Covered stent ☐

A) Polytrauma, unstable in theatre with short mid-SFA disruption with threatened limb identified during external fixator of femoral fracture

B) Explant infected AAA graft

C) Critical limb ischaemia for femoro-distal bypass

D) Redo lower limb bypass for tissue loss with no leg vein available

E) Interposition graft for common femoral aneurysm repair – elective

F) Ligation and debridement of infected false aneurysm EIA in drug user

Question 17

1) Rivaroxaban ☐

2) Low molecular weight heparin ☐

3) Clopidogrel ☐

4) Apixaban ☐

5) Dual antiplatelet therapy ☐

6) Prasugrel ☐

7) Ticlopidine ☐

8) Warfarin ☐

Which of the above medications would be considered the single best agent in the following situations?

A) 38-year-old female with lower limb DVT following prolonged period of travel and inactivity

B) 74-year-old male with lower limb DVT with metastatic cancer

C) 64-year-old female with AF who has undergone a brachial embolectomy and is ready for discharge

D) Following drug eluting stent deployment into the superficial femoral artery

E) Secondary cardiovascular risk reduction in patients with claudication

F) Long-term anticoagulant following heparin-induced thrombocytopenia

Question 18

1) Standard endovascular aneurysm repair ☐
2) Iliac branch graft ☐
3) Open tube graft repair ☐
4) Aortobifemoral bypass ☐
5) Axillobifemoral bypass ☐
6) Covered stent ☐
7) Fenestrated endovascular aneurysm repair ☐
8) Frozen elephant trunk ☐
9) None ☐

Select the most likely treatment option for each of the following situations:

A) NAAASP 58mm infrarenal AAA, low-risk cardiopulmonary exercise testing

B) Non-flow limiting dissection of common iliac artery following cardiac PCI

C) Occlusive distal aorto-iliac disease with critical limb ischaemia

D) 92-year-old male with type IV abdominal aortic aneurysm with unstable angina

E) 72-year-old male juxtarenal abdominal aortic aneurysm with hostile abdomen

Question 19

1) Transfusion related acute lung injury ☐
2) Ventilator associated pneumonia ☐
3) Abdominal compartment syndrome ☐
4) Metformin induced lactate acidosis ☐
5) Coeliac mesenteric ischaemia ☐
6) SMA mesenteric ischaemia ☐
7) Left colonic ischaemia ☐
8) Adhesional bowel obstruction ☐

What is the most likely diagnosis in the following scenarios?

A) Open repair rAAA without autologous blood transfusion, progressive tachypnea, fever, cyanosis and hypotension without signs of heart failure or volume overload

B) rEVAR performed under local anaesthetic; 14 hours later progressive hypotension and desaturation with raised ventilator pressures

C) 70-year-old male with untreated AF who presented with severe abdominal pain without clinical findings and bowel emptying; a D-dimer returns as raised but with normal lactate; subsequently, pain increases and is associated with clinical deterioration and progression towards peritonitis

D) Elective EVAR with left internal iliac embolism and extension to the external iliac performed 5 days earlier; patient presents with abdominal pain, raised D-dimer and bowel opening

Question 20

A) In-patient transfer ☐

B) Urgent vascular clinic appointment within 2 weeks ☐

C) Urgent vascular clinic appointment within 6 weeks ☐

D) Routine vascular clinic appointment ☐

E) Discharge ☐

What is the most appropriate management for each of the following scenarios:

1) 4.5cm asymptomatic AAA found on screening

2) 3.2cm asymptomatic AAA found incidentally on CT KUB

3) 76-year-old male under investigation for pancreatitis identified 5.4cm AAA with retroperitoneal inflammatory changes on imaging

4) 6.2cm AAA in a 67-year-old man found on screening

5) 5.8cm AAA in a 59-year-old woman with back pain

Mr Anthony Thaventhiran
MBBS MRCS
General Surgical Registrar
KSS Deanery

Mr Declan McDonnell
MBBS MRCS
General Surgical Registrar
KSS Deanery

Question 1

A 20-year-old male was admitted via HEMS following a road traffic collision. On scene he looked pale with a thready radial pulse; a ROTEM was run that indicated the patient was coagulopathic. What has been indicated as one of the key drivers of endogenous acute traumatic coagulopathy (ATC)?

    A) Activated protein C

    B) Protein C

    C) Protein S

    D) Von Willebrand's factor

    E) Neutrophils

Question 2

A 27-year-old female cyclist was involved in a road traffic collision with a heavy goods vehicle. On scene her legs were trapped by one of the wheels of the vehicle and the HEMS doctor suspects she could be bleeding from a pelvic injury. A REBOA was inserted at the road side with the balloon inflated and the patient transported via air ambulance to the nearest major trauma centre after extraction. Where should a Zone 3 REBOA be located?

A) Descending thoracic aorta

B) Below the diaphragm and above the renal arteries

C) Below the renal arteries at the point of bifurcation of the aorta

D) Common iliac bifurcation

E) None of the above

Question 3

The above patient was not given tranexamic acid at the prehospital or within the emergency department. The hospital missed out on the best practice tariff from NHS England. A departmental review was instigated after this occurred to a number of patients. When does the CRASH-2 trial recommend tranexamic acid be given?

A) Ideally within 3 hours of the injury but potentially detrimental after 8 hours

B) Ideally within 2 hours of the injury but potentially detrimental after 4 hours

C) Ideally within 30 minutes of the injury but potentially detrimental after 2 hours

D) Ideally within 1 hour of the injury but potentially detrimental after 3 hours

E) Ideally within 2 hours of the injury but potentially detrimental after 6 hours

Question 4

A 17-year-old male was admitted with a single incised wound in the left flank. He was rushed by 'friends' to hospital and dumped at the entrance of the emergency department. He was rushed into Resus and a CT scan confirmed a 2.5cm laceration through the lower pole of the left kidney, with a large surrounding retroperitoneal haematoma and multiple blushes of contract in keeping with an arterial injury. On delayed phase imaging there is a hyperdensity in keeping with a caliceal injury. According to the American Association for the Surgery of Trauma (AAST), what grade of injury has the patient suffered?

A) I

B) II

C) III

D) IV

E) V

Question 5

How should the above patient be managed?

 A) Review by a urologist in the morning

 B) Nephrectomy

 C) Percutaneous embolisation of the left renal artery branch supplying the inferior pole

 D) Antibiotics and admission for close monitoring

 E) Trans-urethral electrocauterisation

Question 6

A builder fell through a skylight, falling 8 feet onto a concrete floor. He was seen by HEMS and had a GCS of 3. He was intubated and transferred by air ambulance to the local major trauma centre, receiving 4 units of whole blood in the 15-minute flight time. On admission to the ED, he had a BP of 59/38, an HR of 120 and fresh blood actively coming from the mouth. A CT scan of his body and head indicates a severe comminuted fracture of the lateral and medial walls of both orbits and both orbital floors as well as the orbital roof, more marked on the left. There are bilateral retrobulbar haematomas, more marked on the left, bilateral proptosis of the globes, and both optic nerves appear to be under a degree of tension. There is a comminuted fracture of the mandible bilaterally including comminuted fracture displacement of the condylar neck and coronoid process.

The OMFS registrar is fast bleeped to Resus. What does the trauma team leader tell them?

 A) Apologise they meant to fast bleep the neurosurgical registrar

 B) Tracheostomy

 C) Decompressive craniectomies

 D) Pack the mouth and lateral canthotomy

 E) Review Le Fort fractures

Question 7

The above patient has a CT Head, which shows an extradural haematoma in the right middle cranial fossa opposed to a subdural haematoma likely secondary to trauma to the right sphenoparietal sinus associated with fractures of the greater wing of the sphenoid on the side. A retroclival subdural haematoma is demonstrated as well as a subarachnoid haemorrhage within the basal cisterns. Generalised cerebral oedema and loss of grey-white differentiation. Clinically he has bilateral blown pupils and shows no improvement despite infusion with mannitol (hypertonic saline). What does the neurosurgical registrar recommend?

A) ICP bolt, remain intubated and transfer to ITU

B) Bifrontal decompressive craniectomies

C) Burr hole

D) Extubate, one hourly neuro-observations, and admit under the general surgeons with a repeat CT scan in the morning

E) Palliation

Question 8

The Trauma Audit and Research Network (TARN) records the Injury Severity Score (ISS), with all injuries assigned an Abbreviated Injury Scale (AIS) code. Patients with multiple injuries are scored by adding together:

A) The 3 highest AIS scores

B) The 4 highest AIS scores

C) The square of the 3 highest AIS scores

D) The square of the 4 highest AIS scores

E) The square root of the 2 highest AIS scores

Question 9

A 15 year old is stabbed in the chest and an ED department thoracotomy is performed. A tamponade of the heart is evacuated and a hole in the atrial appendage closed. Some report an emergency thoracotomy survival for a penetrating injury at 9–12% with some institutions reporting up to 38%. Whilst for blunt trauma on the other hand a survival rate following cardiac arrest is only reported as:

A) 0%

B) 1–2%

C) 5–9%

D) 17%

E) 25%

Question 10

A 20-year-old male is stabbed in the countryside in the right upper quadrant and rushed into the local district general hospital as he is too unstable to make to it to the local major trauma centre. A major haemorrhage protocol is activated and damage control resuscitation (DCR) is started whilst the theatre is being prepped for damage control surgery (DCS). Unfortunately, the only CT scanner is being repaired. The on-call general surgeon is a specialist in pelvic floor dysfunction but has recently just returned from a DSTS course. What should they do in theatre?

A) Pack the abdomen and in particular try to control the liver, and transfer to the local MTC if the patient remains unstable

B) Thoracotomy and cross clamp the descending thoracic aorta and transfer to the local MTC

C) Hepatectomy of the affected lobe of the liver

D) Cattell-Braasch manoeuvre and deal with the affected organs

E) Ask the interventional radiologist to embolise the affected segment of the liver

Question 11

What is the definition of a massive transfusion?

A) >10 units of blood products within 24 hours

B) >10 units of blood products within 1 hour

C) >10 units of blood products within 6 hours

D) >4 units of blood products within 1 hour

E) >4 units of blood products within 30 minutes

Question 12

A 16-year-old boy is stabbed outside his school and has an arterial-looking spray coming from his leg. HEMs attend and place a tourniquet and haemostatic gauze over the wound and administer tranexamic acid and two units of whole blood. He is rushed into the local major trauma centre where a major haemorrhage protocol/code red is activated. At admission a ROTEM is run that shows in EXTEM, the LI 30 (Lysis Index after 30 minutes) is less than 85%. What should be given immediately to treat the hyperfibrinolysis?

A) Cryoprecipitate

B) Platelets

C) Plasma

D) Tranexamic acid

E) Packed red cells

Question 13

Having fallen off a horse and been trampled, a patient is admitted with a haemopneumothorax. A chest drain is inserted. In what anatomical place should this ideally be placed?

A) Posterior to the midaxillary line over the fifth intercostal rib

B) Anterior to the midaxillary line below the fifth intercostal rib

C) Anterior to the midaxillary line over the fifth intercostal rib

D) Posterior to the midaxillary line over the fifth intercostal rib

E) Mid clavicular line below the third intercostal space

Extended Matching Question 14 – Trauma Techniques

A) Kocher manoeuvre ☐

B) Mattox manoeuvre ☐

C) Cattell–Braasch manoeuvre ☐

D) Conservative ☐

E) Pringle manoeuvre ☐

F) Left anterolateral thoracotomy ☐

G) Right posterolateral thoracotomy ☐

H) Clamshell thoracotomy ☐

I) Pericardiocentesis ☐

J) Pre-peritoneal packing ☐

Match the appropriate option from the above list with each of the following:

1) Expose the infrarenal IVC

2) Manage a supramesocolic haematoma

3) Visualise the pancreatic head

4) Reduce bleeding from the liver

5) Evacuate cardiac tamponade

6) Access a lacerated pulmonary trunk

7) Control bleeding from a pelvic fracture when angiography unavailable

8) Manage a blunt perinephric haematoma

Extended Matching Question 15 – Burns

A) Wallace ☐

B) Parkland ☐

C) Lund & Browder ☐

D) Palmer ☐

E) Superficial ☐

F) Superficial partial thickness ☐

G) Deep dermal ☐

H) Full thickness ☐

I) Jackson ☐

J) Curreri ☐

Match the appropriate option from the above list with each of the following:

1) Eponymous "Rule of Nines" used to assess the extent of burn injuries

2) Eponymous technique that uses the patient's palm size to assess the extent of burns

3) The most accurate method for establishing the true extent of burns

4) The most used method of determining volume of fluid needed for resuscitation

5) Burn depth only involving the epidermis

6) Burn depth characterised by pain, small blister formation and hyperaemia

7) Burn producing an insensate, waxy or leathery appearance of skin

8) Blotchy red appearance with significant risk of hypertrophic scarring

Extended Matching Question 16 – Trauma Figures

A) 5 ☐

B) 10 ☐

C) 15 ☐

D) 20 ☐

E) 30 ☐

F) 40 ☐

G) 50 ☐

H) 75 ☐

I) 100 ☐

J) 150 ☐

Match the appropriate option from the above list with each of the following:

1) What percentage of the cardiac index is produced by external chest compressions?

2) What percentage of the cardiac index is produced by internal chest compressions?

3) The percentage surface area with a subcapsular haematoma in grade I splenic trauma

4) The percentage surface area with a subcapsular haematoma in grade III hepatic trauma

5) The maximum Injury Severity Score

6) The maximum Glasgow Coma Score

7) Circulating blood loss less than this percentage corresponds to grade I haemorrhagic shock

8) Circulating blood loss greater than this percentage corresponds to grade IV haemorrhagic shock

9) What percentage of blunt trauma is due to falls in the UK?

10) What percentage of blunt trauma is due to motor vehicle collisions in the UK?

CHAPTER 17
BARIATRIC SURGERY

Answers on page 298–302

Ms Jihène El Kafsi
MA FRCS
Consultant UGI Surgeon, Frimley Health NHS Foundation Trust

Mr Naim Fakih Gomez
MD FRCS
Consultant Bariatric Surgeon, University College London Hospital

Question 1

What is Petersen's defect in a Roux-en-Y gastric bypass?

A) Port site hernia defect

B) Space between two edges of small bowel mesentery

C) Space between transverse colonic mesentery and biliary limb small bowel mesentery

D) Space between transverse colonic mesentery and alimentary limb small bowel mesentery

E) The defect created in the colonic mesentery in a retrocolic gastric bypass

Question 2

Which of the following is a contraindication to a sleeve gastrectomy?

A) Barrett's oesophagus

B) Hiatus hernia

C) Previous abdominal surgery

D) Crohn's disease

E) Familial adenomatous polyposis

Question 3

Which of these is an absolute contraindication to bariatric surgery?

A) Type 1 diabetes mellitus

B) Crohn's disease

C) Cardiac failure

D) Active untreated psychiatric illness

E) Age over 65

Question 4

A 46-year-old smoker with a history of a gastric bypass performed 4 years ago presents to ED with severe epigastric pain, temperature 38 and tachycardia. What is the most likely diagnosis?

A) Pancreatitis

B) Biliary colic

C) Gastric ulcer

D) Gastrojejunal ulcer perforation

E) Gastrojejunal ulcer bleed

Question 5

What is the next most appropriate investigation?

A) CT abdomen with oral contrast

B) Contrast swallow

C) USS of liver and gallbladder

D) Diagnostic laparoscopy

E) OGD

Question 6

At laparoscopy there is a perforation at the gastrojejunal anastomosis. The most appropriate next step is:

A) Gastrojejunal anastomosis resection and redo

B) Washout and drains

C) Primary repair

D) Omental patch repair

E) Serosal patch repair

Question 7

A 33-year-old woman with a previous gastric bypass is admitted to hospital confused and dishevelled. She has a BMI of 18. History from a relative reveals that she has not been taking multivitamins and has a history of alcohol abuse. Which vitamin deficiency must be suspected?

    A) Vitamin D

    B) Vitamin B3

    C) Vitamin B12

    D) Vitamin B1

    E) All of the above

Question 8

What is the next step in suspected thiamine deficiency?

    A) Urgent serum thiamine level

    B) Oral thiamine replacement

    C) IV thiamine replacement

    D) Parenteral nutrition

    E) All of the above

Question 9

What is Wernicke's classic triad?

    A) Ophthalmoplegia, cerebellar dysfunction, confusion

    B) Confusion, dermatitis, diarrhoea

    C) Dermatitis, diarrhoea and dementia

    D) Hair loss, paraesthesia and gum bleeding

    E) Fatigue, anaemia and heart failure

Question 10

Which of the following nutritional deficiencies might develop in the first six months after a derivative bariatric procedure?

A) Bilateral sensorial and motor polyneuropathy caused by vitamin B1 deficiency

B) Bilateral sensorial and motor polyneuropathy caused by vitamin B12 deficiency

C) Bilateral sensorial and motor polyneuropathy caused by folate deficiency

D) Bilateral sensorial and motor polyneuropathy caused by folate and vitamin B12 deficiency

E) All of the above

Question 11

Which of these patients fit NICE criteria and do not have contraindications for bariatric surgery?

A) BMI 32 Caucasian with HbA1c 38

B) BMI 29 Asian with HbA1c 50

C) BMI 37 Asian with no comorbidities

D) BMI 38 Caucasian with no comorbidities

E) None of the above

Question 12

Which of these patients fit NICE criteria and do not have contraindications for bariatric surgery?

A) BMI 45 Caucasian with obstructive sleep apnoea

B) BMI 34 Asian with type 2 diabetes

C) BMI 40 Afro-Caribbean no comorbidities

D) BMI 32 Caucasian with new onset type 2 diabetes

E) All of the above

Question 13

Which of these patients fit NICE criteria and do not have contraindications for bariatric surgery?

    A) BMI 45 with T2DM with a slipped gastric band

    B) BMI 35 with T2DM schizophrenic with suicide attempt 2 months ago

    C) BMI 40 with new diagnosis of colon cancer

    D) BMI 40 with total colectomy for UC and Barrett's oesophagus

    E) None of the above

Question 14

A 45-year-old male had an adjustable gastric band inserted 3 years ago. His preoperative BMI was 41 kg/m2 and did not present any comorbidities. He had regular follow-up and adjustments in the band clinic in a bariatric surgery unit, and currently has 8 mls in the band out of an original 10 mls. Patient lost 22 kg. The patient presents to A&E with daily vomiting and nausea after a week of flu-like symptoms. All of this should be considered except:

    A) Gastritis or peptic duodenitis

    B) Band slippage

    C) Intragastric migration

    D) Marginal ulceration

    E) All of the above should be considered

Question 15

The above patient's GP treated him with omeprazole 20 mg od and indicated a liquid diet. The patient was referred to you for a barium swallow. Which of the following is NOT present?

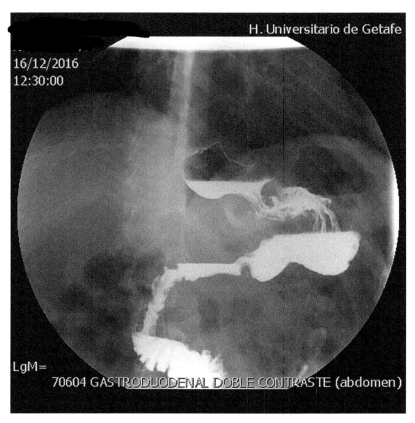

A) Hiatal hernia with a dilated pouch

B) Band slippage

C) Perforation at the gastric pouch

D) "O" sign

E) All of the above are present

Question 16

Which initial management step is most appropriate given this diagnosis?

- A) Discharge on omeprazole to 20 mg bd, oral antiemetics and prokinetics
- B) Laparoscopic hiatal hernia repair
- C) Conservative management: NG tube insertion, IV fluid therapy and bowel rest
- D) NBM, IV fluid therapy and aspiration of the band port
- E) None of the above

Extended Matching Question 17

- A) Roux en Y gastric bypass ☐
- B) One anastomosis gastric bypass ☐
- C) Sleeve gastrectomy ☐
- D) Adjustable gastric band ☐
- E) Duodenal switch ☐
- F) Biliopancreatic diversion ☐
- G) Single anastomosis duodeno-ileal bypass (SADI) ☐
- H) Gastric plication ☐

Match an appropriate option from the above list with each of the following:

1) Duodenoileostomy and 1 mesenteric defect
2) Most common bariatric procedure worldwide
3) Perigastric technique
4) Antireflux procedure
5) Distal gastrectomy
6) Billroth type 2 gastrojejunostomy
7) Gastrogastric herniation (complication)
8) Duodenoileostomy and 2 mesenteric defects

Extended Matching Question 18 – Complications and Procedure

A) Duodenal stump leak ☐

B) Jejunojenunostomy intussusception ☐

C) 'Corkscrew' twist ☐

D) Gastrogastric herniation ☐

E) Intragastric migration ☐

F) Bile reflux ☐

G) Staple line disruption with weight regain ☐

Match an appropriate option from the above list with each of the following:

1) Sleeve gastrectomy

2) Adjustable gastric band

3) Roux en Y gastric bypass

4) One anastomosis gastric bypass

5) Single anastomosis duodeno-ileal bypass (SADI)

6) Vertical banded gastroplasty

7) Gastric plication

Extended Matching Question 19 – Procedure of Choice

A) Male, 57 years, Caucasian, non-smoker, severe GORD, BMI 43 ☐

B) Female, 24 years, Caucasian, smoker, BMI 47 ☐

C) Male, 37 years, Asian, non-smoker, BMI 29, T2DM on metformin ☐

D) Female, 48 years, Asian, non-smoker, BMI 33, depression ☐

E) Female, 42 years, Caucasian, non-smoker, BMI 41; eroded gastric band in situ ☐

F) Male, 32 years, Caucasian, non-smoker, BMI 28; previous sleeve gastrectomy; significant GORD non-responsive to medical treatment ☐

G) Female, 39 years, Asian, non-smoker, BMI 44; previous adjustable gastric band; leak in tubing system and failure to lose weight ☐

Match an appropriate option from the above list with each of the following:

1) One stage: band removal and revisional RYGB

2) Revision Roux en Y gastric bypass

3) Primary Roux en Y gastric bypass (RYGB)

4) Sleeve gastrectomy / RYGB

5) Two stage: band removal and revisional RYGB

6) Sleeve gastrectomy

7) Non-surgical weight management programme

Miss Prizzi Zarsadias
BSc MBChB MRCS
General Surgical Registrar
East Kent Hospital University Foundation Trust

Miss Disha Mehta
MBBS BSc MRCS
Specialist Registrar in General Surgery
Kent, Surrey and Sussex Deanery

Mr Chinedu Chianakwalam
MBBS FRCSI MSc
Consultant Breast and General Surgeon
East Kent Hospital University Foundation Trust

Question 1

A 38-year-old premenopausal patient has a grade 2 25mm invasive ductal carcinoma right breast cancer for which she has undergone wide local excision and sentinel node biopsy. The tumour is ER negative, PR negative, HER2 positive. She is node negative and margins are clear. What is the next step in management?

- A) Focal breast radiotherapy followed by tamoxifen for at least 5 years
- B) Axillary node clearance, radiotherapy for whole breast followed by chemotherapy and trastuzumab
- C) Adjuvant chemotherapy and trastuzumab followed by whole breast radiotherapy
- D) Discuss mastectomy and reconstruction options
- E) Commence anastrozole for minimum 5 years

Question 2

A 23 year old has been referred to the one-stop breast clinic with a palpable mobile left breast lump that has been present for 3 months. It has caused intermittent discomfort, usually coinciding with the beginning of her period. She has not had a lump before. She is fit and healthy otherwise and takes the oral contraceptive pill. She has no relevant family history. She has an ultrasound demonstrating a well-circumscribed ovoid lesion that is 2.2cm with features of a fibroadenoma. What is the next step?

A) Wide local excision and discharge following confirmation of histology and clear margins

B) Reassure the patient; excision is not necessary; the patient can be safely discharged

C) Discussion at MDT, urgent excision and recommendation to immediately stop oral contraceptive medication

D) Urgent core biopsy followed by excision

E) Arrange an interval ultrasound of breast in 6 months; recommend excision if lesion has increased in size

Question 3

A 38-year-old male patient attends clinic with increased volume of breast tissue. He takes no medication. Part of his work up included blood tests. These have demonstrated normal renal, liver and thyroid function. He undergoes endocrine testing and is found to have low leutinising hormone, low testosterone and raised prolactin. What is the cause for his symptoms?

A) Pituitary adenoma

B) Primary hypogonadism

C) Testicular cancer

D) Adrenal neoplasm

E) Breast malignancy

Question 4

Tamoxifen has been commenced on a 51 year old diagnosed with 18mm grade 2 invasive ductal carcinoma of the right breast, node negative, receptor status ER + PR - HER2-. She has been taking the medication for 18 months and has ceased to have periods for the past year. She attends the breast clinic for her annual follow up and clinical exam demonstrates no sign of recurrence. What investigation(s) should be requested?

A) Breast MRI

B) FSH, bHCG, thyroid function

C) Ca 125 and transvaginal ultrasound

D) Mammogram and FSH

E) CT chest abdo pelvis and targeted breast ultrasound

Question 5

A patient has undergone triple assessment of a lump. Biopsy showed a fibroepithelial lesion and the differential diagnosis is between a phyllodes tumour and a cellular fibroadenoma. How should it be treated?

A) Reassure the patient that a phyllodes tumour is entirely benign; excision is not necessary; the patient can be safely discharged

B) Following MDT discussion, patients should undergo excisional biopsy

C) Urgent mastectomy followed by radiotherapy

D) Repeat imaging in 6 months

E) Wide local excision and sentinel node biopsy

Question 6

With regard to nipple discharge, which of the following is true?

A) 55% of nipple discharge is associated with malignancy

B) Nipple smear cytology has a sensitivity of 11.1–16.7%

C) Benign intraductal papillomas present with clear discharge

D) Thyroid function tests are not indicated in the investigation of nipple discharge

E) Colour of nipple discharge is a reliable method of distinguishing between physiological, benign and malignant nipple discharge

Question 7

The following are true for adjuvant radiotherapy in breast cancer, except:

A) Post-operative radiotherapy reduces the risk of ipsilateral recurrence in patients with DCIS, as well as the development of invasive carcinoma

B) The absolute benefit of adjuvant radiotherapy in low risk, small (<2cm), well-differentiated, hormone receptor-positive tumours is small

C) The overall impact of adjuvant radiotherapy is a 23% reduction of any first recurrence

D) All patients should be considered for a breast boost and whole breast irradiation

E) Three-dimensional planning, as well as breath holding, has reduced cardiac irradiation in left-sided tumours

Question 8

With regard to the genetics of breast cancer, which of the following is true?

A) Approximately 7–8% of breast cancer is due to the inheritance of a high penetrance, autosomal dominant, cancer predisposing gene

B) BRCA genes are linked to an increased incidence of adrenal tumours

C) A risk-reduction mastectomy is associated with an 100% reduction in risk

D) In women who have established unilateral breast cancer, there is a 1–2% risk of having cancer in the contralateral breast

E) The Ashkenazi Jewish population has three founder mutations within the BRCA genes, which are found in 2% of their population

Question 9

When considering molecular tumour markers, the following are true, except:

A) Human epidermal growth factor receptor 2 is a cell surface tyrosine kinase receptor-like molecule, regulating cell growth and differentiation

B) 36–39% of breast cancers overexpress this protein

C) It is associated with a poor prognosis

D) Tumours are classified as HER-2 positive if they score 3+ on immunohistochemical staining, or are positive on fluorescent in-situ hybridisation (FiSH)

E) Adjuvant therapy with Trastuzumab carries a risk of cardiotoxicity, reducing left ventricular function by 4%, at 2–3 years

Question 10

The following statements regarding axillary surgery are true, except:

A) Involved axillary lymph nodes with invasive breast disease on preoperative ultrasound and biopsy warrants an axillary clearance

B) An FNA pre-operatively showing normal lymph-node cells warrants a sentinel lymph-node biopsy

C) Sentinel lymph-node biopsy is associated with an increased risk of lymphoedema, reduced mobility and paraesthesia

D) When performing a mastectomy for DCIS, axillary surgery in any form does not need to be considered

E) Axillary node dissection is not associated with improved survival in sentinel node positive patients

Question 11

With regard to breast screening, which of the following is true?

A) High-grade DCIS is one of the most important cancers to be detected at screening

B) Women are invited for a two-view mammogram, every 2 years from the age of 49

C) Approximately 8% of screened women are recalled for further assessment

D) False positive recall and benign surgical biopsy are more likely in older women

E) NICE guidelines recommend annual MRI surveillance for women aged 30–39 with a 10-year risk of >5%

Extended Matching Question 12

A) Mammogram and US breast ☐

B) US breast ☐

C) Clinical biopsy ☐

D) Stereotatic mammogram biopsy ☐

E) MRI breast ☐

F) Urgent wide local excision and sentinel-node biopsy ☐

G) US and biopsy ☐

H) Scope major ducts ☐

I) Major duct excision ☐

From the above options, select the most appropriate next step for the following scenarios:

1) A 45-year-old patient attends one-stop breast clinic and has a density picked up on mammogram but not on ultrasound. She is re-examined and her clinical examination demonstrates a suspicious P3 lesion.

2) Following a workplace health screen, a 38-year-old patient was found to have interderminate micro calcification on mammogram. She attends the outpatient clinic – her past medical history, family history and clinical examination is unremarkable.

3) A 51-year-old patient has persistent bloody nipple discharge. Mammogram and US of the subareolar tissue is normal.

4) A 40-year-old patient attends clinic with change in the contour of her breasts. She has bilateral silicone implants.

5) During annual follow-up clinic, a 47 year old points out a change in her wide local excision scar which has localised thickening.

6) A patient re-attends one-stop breast clinic. She had a normal mammogram 8 months ago for a breast lump that, after triple assessment, is diagnosed with fibroadenoma. She has a new lump.

CHAPTER 19
ENDOCRINE
SURGERY

Answers on page 306–313

Mr Veera J. Allu

MS ChM FRCS (Gen Surg)
General and Emergency Surgeon
East Kent Hospital University Foundation Trust

Question 1

Regarding primary hyperparathyroidism (PHP), the most common presenting clinical finding is:

  A) Bone pain

  B) Fatigue

  C) Renal calculi

  D) GI symptoms related to PUD or pancreatitis

  E) Asymptomatic

Question 2

The commonest cause for PHP is:

  A) Adenoma

  B) Double adenoma

  C) Hyperplasia

  D) Carcinoma

  E) Both B and C

Question 3

Regarding PHP, which of the following is the least sensitive in the pre-operative localisation of abnormal parathyroid gland?

A) Single photon emission CT(SPECT)

B) MRI

C) Standard CT

D) Ultrasound of the neck

E) Sestamibi scan

Question 4

A 52-year-old lady presented to A&E with increasing confusion, vomiting, generalised weakness and anxiety. Blood picture showed chronic renal failure along with highly elevated serum calcium levels. What's the immediate management plan?

A) Biphosphonates

B) Immediate frusemide infusion

C) Emergency parathyroidectomy

D) Intravenous fluid hydration

E) Infusion of calcitonin

Question 5

With regard to routine work up for PHP, all of the following are included except:

A) 24-hour urinary calcium estimation

B) Serum calcium levels

C) Intact PTH (iPTH)

D) Serum 1,25-dihydroxyvitamin D levels

E) Chloride : phosphate ratio

Question 6

All of the following conditions can cause hypercalcaemia in patients with normal parathyroid function except:

A) Malignancy

B) Lithium

C) Sarcoidosis

D) Vitamin D intoxication

E) Cirrhosis

Question 7

A patient had minimally invasive parathyroidectomy (MIP) for PHP 6 months ago. He is still symptomatic. Where would be the commonest location for a missed parathyroid adenoma in patients undergoing re-operation for parathyroid surgery?

A) Thymus

B) Carotid sheath

C) Tracheoesophageal groove

D) Superior pole of the thyroid

E) Further low in the mediastinum

Question 8

A patient had a CT scan of abdomen for non-specific abdominal pain. There was an incidental finding of an adrenal mass measuring 3cm. The appropriate next step in the management of this finding would be:

A) Observation

B) CT-guided FNAC

C) Laparoscopic adrenalectomy

D) Bio-chemical workup

E) Thyroid and parathyroid profile

Question 9

A 45-year-old lady is on the waiting list to undergo laparoscopic adrenalectomy for a pheochromocytoma. Which of the following agents should not be used as the initial medication to achieve the appropriate preoperative adrenoreceptor blockade?

A) Phenoxybenzamine

B) Epinephrine with incremental doses of norepinephrine

C) Prazosin

D) Atenolol

E) Amlodipine

Question 10

Which of the following is not an associated feature of Cushing syndrome?

A) Hypernatraemia

B) Hyperkalaemia

C) Psychosis

D) Hyperglycaemia

E) Increased levels of cortisol

Question 11

The commonest cause of Cushing syndrome is:

A) Pituitary adenoma

B) Adrenal adenoma

C) Adrenal hyperplasia

D) Ectopic secretion

E) Steroids

Question 12

With regards to thyroid anatomy, which of the following statements is incorrect?

A) The superior thyroid artery arises directly from the thyrocervical trunk and passes upward in front of the vertebral artery

B) The thyroid ima artery arises directly from the aorta in <5% of patients

C) The superior and middle thyroid veins drain into the internal jugular vein

D) Venous drainage of the thyroid gland is via the superior, middle and inferior branches

E) The superior and inferior thyroid arteries join behind the outer part of the thyroid lobes

Question 13

Measurement of calcitonin is essential in what disease process?

A) Papillary thyroid cancer

B) Follicular thyroid cancer

C) Medullary thyroid cancer

D) Anaplastic carcinoma

E) Lymphoma of the thyroid

Question 14

A 40-year-old woman complains of anxiety, irritability, heat intolerance, along with weight loss. On examination, she has a small palpable nodule on the right side of her neck close to the midline. Her laboratory work up revealed suppressed TSH levels. What is the next step in the management of this patient?

A) Radioactive iodine scan

B) FNAC

C) Ultrasound neck

D) MRI

E) CT

Question 15

In a case of Grave's disease, pre-operative preparation should include all the following except:

A) Anti-thyroid drugs

B) Lugol's iodine

C) High-dose cholestyramine

D) β blockers

E) Lithium

Question 16

A patient presented with 2cm nodule located on his left thyroid lobe. FNAC revealed THY3. What is the next appropriate step in the management of this patient?

    A) Lobectomy

    B) Subtotal thyroidectomy

    C) Total thyroidectomy

    D) Repeat FNAC

    E) Close observation every 3 months

Question 17

Which of the following is not considered to be an increased risk factor for thyroid cancer in a patient with thyroid mass?

    A) Young age

    B) Male gender

    C) Family history

    D) Neck irradiation during childhood

    E) Hot nodule on iodine scan

Question 18

Which is the most common malignancy of the thyroid?

    A) Papillary

    B) Follicular

    C) Medullary

    D) Anaplastic

    E) Hurtle cell carcinoma

Question 19

With regard to differentiated thyroid cancers, which is considered the most important prognostic factor in thyroid staging systems?

    A) Size

    B) Nodal status

    C) Age

    D) Grading

    E) Extrathyroidal spread

Question 20

A 30-year-old man presented with a thyroid nodule along with elevated levels of calcitonin. Regarding further management, all are acceptable apart from:

    A) Genetic counselling to family members

    B) CEA is a useful marker

    C) Total thyroidectomy

    D) Biochemical workup

    E) Ultrasound of the neck to check on lymph-node status

Question 21

A 70-year-old woman has been experiencing fevers, night sweats and weight loss for a few months. She was on regular thyroxine replacement for many years. Examination of her neck found a palpable mass that was tender. U/S revealed a 3–4cm right thyroid mass and FNAC is non-diagnostic. What is the next step in the management of this patient?

    A) Radioactive iodine scan

    B) Anti-tuberculous treatment

    C) NSAID

    D) Repeat FNAC under U/S guidance

    E) Open biopsy

Question 22

Regarding insulinomas, all the following are true except:

    A) They arise from beta-cell of the pancreas

    B) Usually benign lesions

    C) Unifocal

    D) Serum calcium levels may be elevated

    E) Should be screened for MEN2

Question 23

What is the risk of recurrent laryngeal nerve injury during routine thyroid surgery?

    A) <1%

    B) <2%

    C) <3%

    D) <4%

    E) 5–10%

Question 24

Regarding pheochromocytoma, which is the best technique to localise the lesion?

    A) Sestamabi scan

    B) MIBG scan

    C) SPECT

    D) MRI with contrast

    E) Colour duplex scan

Question 25

Multiple endocrine neoplasia II includes all the following except:

    A) Medullary thyroid cancer

    B) Pheochromocytoma

    C) Hyperparathyroidism

    D) Mucosal neuromas

    E) Islet cell tumours of pancreas

Question 26

In a thyroidectomy, the following are all anatomical regions in which the recurrent laryngeal nerve is commonly found except:

    A) Tracheoesophageal groove

    B) Crossing the inferior thyroid artery

    C) Anterior to the inferior thyroid artery

    D) Posterior to the tuberculum Zuckerkandl

    E) Anterior to the tuberculum Zuckerkandl

Question 27

The incidence of hypocalcaemia post thyroidectomy as defined by the British Association of Endocrine and Thyroid Surgeons (BAETS) registry on the fourth UK national audit was found to be:

A) 2.7%

B) 6.3%

C) 15.2%

D) 24.9%

E) 37.1%

Question 28

Which form of thyroid malignancy secretes the tumour marker calcitonin?

A) Medullary

B) Follicular

C) Anaplastic

D) Lymphoma

E) Metastases to the thyroid

Question 29

Which of the following statements is true with regard to adrenal tumours?

A) Mostly incidentalomas

B) Adrenal metastases are more common than primary adrenal cortical cancer

C) Local invasion is a suspicious radiographic finding

D) Non-contrast CT attenuation greater than 10 Hounsfield units is a suspicious radiographic finding

E) all of the above

Question 30

What is the most common adrenal tumour found by incidentalomas?

A) Cushing's adenoma

B) Non-functioning adenoma

C) Adrenocortical carcinoma

D) Metastases

E) Phaeochromocytoma

Question 31

Typically what colour are parathyroid glands?

A) Sunset orange

B) Gunmetal grey

C) Moon white

D) Portland brick

E) Autumn brown

Question 32

Where does the blood supply of the superior parathyroid gland usually arise?

A) Inferior thyroid artery

B) Superior thyroid artery

C) Thyroid ima

D) All of the above

E) None of the above

CHAPTER 20
TRANSPLANT SURGERY

Answers on page 313–316

Mr Rupesh Sutaria
BSc (Hons), MBBS, MD, FRCS
Consultant Transplant and General Surgeon
Queen Alexandra Hospital, Portsmouth

Extended Matching Question 1 – Fistula

- A) Ligate fistula ☐
- B) Fistuloplasty ☐
- C) Banding ☐
- D) Brachio-cephalic fistula ☐
- E) Radio-cephalic fistula ☐
- F) Brachio-basilic transposition fistula ☐
- G) Tunnelled line ☐
- H) Non-tunnelled line ☐
- I) Interposition graft ☐
- J) Duplex ☐
- K) Fistulogram ☐

Choose the appropriate option from the above list for each of the following:

1) A 70-year-old diabetic with increasingly cold and painful fingers with a working brachiocephalic fistula

2) A 25-year-old patient requiring access for dialysis with a duplex showing a 3mm cephalic vein at the wrist and 4mm at the elbow; has a 2mm radial artery and 4mm brachial artery

3) A 56-year-old patient with prolonged bleeding after removal of needles from an upper-arm straight PTFE graft

4) A 64-year-old unstable patient with actively bleeding pseudoaneurysm from a brachio-basilic transposition fistula

5) Access type most associated with infections

Question 2 – Brain-dead Donor Criteria

For the diagnosis and confirmation of brain stem death:

A) Death may be confirmed by two experienced registrars registered for more than 5 years

B) Death may be confirmed by two consultants from an organ retrieval team

C) Two set of tests must be performed a minimum of 6 hours apart

D) Spinal reflex movement of a limb excludes a diagnosis of brain stem death

E) The legal time of death is after the completion of the first set of tests that confirm brain stem death

Question 3 – Exclusion to Organ Donation

Which option would not be an absolute contraindication to organ donation?

A) HIV disease

B) Active and untreated TB

C) Completely excised stage 2 melanoma

D) T2N0M0 breast cancer treated 5 years ago

E) Myeloma not currently in remission

Extended Matching Question 4 – Immunosuppression

A) Campath ☐

B) Basliximab ☐

C) Rituximab ☐

D) Methylprednisolone ☐

E) Tacrolimus ☐

F) Mycofenolate ☐

G) Ultrasound ☐

H) CT ☐

I) Biopsy ☐

J)	Retransplant	☐
K)	Embolectomy	☐
L)	Plasma exchange	☐
M)	ATG	☐
N)	PTC	☐
O)	ERCP	☐
P)	Nephrostogram	☐
Q)	Nephrostomy	☐

Choose the appropriate option from the above list for each of the following:

1) A 38-year-old female 10 days post DCD kidney transplant. A biopsy for delayed graft function shows T-cell mediated rejection. The next step to manage the patient would be…

2) A 44-year-old 5 days post DBD liver transplant. Patient becoming coagulopathic, acidiotic and worsening liver function tests. CT angiogram show hepatic artery thrombosis.

3) A 63-year-old 2 days post live donor kidney transplant with primary function has a reduction in urinary output with a normal blood pressure and an unobstructed catheter.

4) A 28-year-old 7 days post simultaneous pancreas and kidney transplant has rising blood sugars.

5) Ultrasound of recently transplanted kidney shows hydronephrosis.

Question 5

A patient on continuous ambulatory peritoneal dialysis presents with abdominal pain and cloudy bags. Culture of the fluid grows candida.

A) Pull PD catheter out

B) IV gentamicin

C) Removal of PD catheter and washout

D) Intra-abdominal vancomycin

E) Oral flucloxacillin

Question 6 – Indication for Pancreas Transplant

Which of the following could be considered for a pancreas transplant?

    A) Diabetic requiring 130 units/day

    B) Insulin dependent Type II diabetic with BMI 25

    C) Myocardial infarction 3 months ago

    D) Diverticular abscess currently with a percutaneous drain

    E) Successfully treated pancreatic cancer treated 10 years ago with no recurrence

Question 7

Which of the following is an inhibitor of inosine monophosphate dehydrogenase?

    A) Tacrolimus

    B) MMF

    C) Prednisolone

    D) Ciclosporin

    E) Basliximab

Question 8

A kidney donor with blood group AB may donate to which of the following blood groups?

    A) A

    B) B

    C) AB

    D) O

    E) All of the above

Question 9

Which of the following could be considered for a liver transplant?

    A) 4 HCC tumours all under 3cm

    B) Single 4cm colorectal metastasis in left lobe

    C) Cholangiocarcinoma

    D) Bilateral colorectal metastasis

    E) Single HCC measuring 8cm

Question 10

Which factors would reduce the quality of a potential deceased kidney donor?

    A) Previous DVT

    B) Death by RTA

    C) Previous history of breast cancer

    D) Cause of death by stroke

    E) Paediatric donor

Question 11

Which of the following would not be a contraindication for a liver transplant?

    A) Patient with alcoholic hepatitis

    B) Patient with end-stage alcohol disease who has been non-compliant at least twice over the past year with medical care

    C) α-fetoprotein (AFP) 3200 iu/ml

    D) Probability of death of 20% from liver disease at 1 year

    E) 8cm HCC with no vascular invasion of metastasis

Question 12

Which of the following elements is not used when allocating deceased kidneys currently?

    A) Blood group

    B) Age mismatch

    C) Weight mismatch

    D) Waiting time

    E) HLA match

Question 13

Regarding HLA, which of the following is true?

    A) HLA DR mismatch has less of an impact on renal graft outcome than HLA A mismatch

    B) HLA class I antigens are only found on antigen presenting cells

    C) HLA are encoded on chromosome 12

    D) HLA genes have only a few alleles

    E) Are not matched prior to liver transplantation

Question 14

Regarding post-transplant malignancy, which of the following is false?

A) With modern immunosuppression transplant recipients are of no higher overall risk of malignancy than the general population

B) Skin cancer is the most commonly observed cancer post transplant

C) PTLD is the most commonly observed cancer post transplant

D) Successful solid organ transplant reduces the risk of malignancy

E) Should aim to maintain current levels of immunosuppression when a malignancy is diagnosed

Question 15

Regarding PTLD, which of the following is true?

A) Usually unrelated to EBV

B) Unrelated to the type of immunosuppression used

C) Rituximab may be used as treatment

D) Is more common in kidney transplant recipients than bowel recipient patients

E) Always presents with graft dysfunction

Question 16

A patient presents with a clotted brachio-cephalic fistula and a potassium of 6.9. The first step in managing this patient would be:

A) Tunnelled line and dialysis

B) Temporary line and dialysis

C) Open thrombectomy under GA

D) Fistulogram

E) IV heparin

Question 17

A renal transplant patient presents with headache and tremor with increase in creatinine. She has been on a course of fluconazole for candida. What do you do?

A) Check tacrolimus levels

B) Biopsy

C) Ultrasound

D) Pulse with steroids

E) Nephrostomy

Question 18

Following a renal transplant biopsy, a patient is BK virus positive. How should this be treated?

A) Increase tacrolimus

B) Oral ciprofloxacin

C) Decrease immunosuppression

D) Pulse with steroids

E) Valganciclovir

Extended Matching Question 19 – Liver Transplant

A) Portal vein thrombosis ☐

B) Hepatic artery thrombosis ☐

C) Small for size ☐

D) Veno-caval stenosis ☐

E) Bile leak ☐

F) Recurrent disease ☐

G) Bleeding ☐

H) Rejection ☐

I) Ischaemic cholangiopathy ☐

J) Delayed graft function ☐

). Primary non-function ☐

Choose the appropriate option from the above list for each of the following:

1) A 44-year-old presents with increasing ascites and lower leg oedema following a DBD liver transplant 7 months earlier.

2) A 55-year-old 3 days post DCD liver transplant with initial function now is febrile with deterioration in liver function test and requiring inotrope support.

3) A 4-year-old 3 days post split liver transplant has an upper GI bleed and mild liver dysfunction.

Miss Maria Satchi
BM, BSc (Hons), FRCS (Urol)
Post CCT Andrology Fellow
University College London Hospitals NHS Foundation Trust

Mr Andrew Chetwood
BMedSci (Hons), MBChB (Hons), FRCS (Urol)
Consultant Urologist, Frimley Health NHS Foundation Trust

Question 1

A 3-year-old boy is seen with a history of an intermittent left scrotal swelling since birth that is gradually getting larger. On examination you are able to reach above the swelling, which trans-illuminates. What is the next step in his management?

    A) Plan for ligation of left patent processus vaginalis

    B) Reassure the parents and continue observation

    C) Plan for repair of left hydrocele via the scrotal approach

    D) Emergency scrotal exploration

    E) Course of oral antibiotics

Question 2

A patient on the ward has gone into acute urinary retention. He has had a previous laparotomy 5 years ago. The surgical CT2 has done a bladder scan that confirms >999ml in the bladder and has failed at urethral catheterisation. You are also unable to insert a urethral catheter. There is no urology cover on site and the patient is in significant pain. What is your next step?

A) Contact urology team at a nearby trust for transfer of the patient

B) Perform a suprapubic catheter insertion on the ward

C) Organise a CT scan

D) Aspirate urine using a 21G needle and syringe

E) Urgent open suprapubic catheter insertion on CEPOD

Question 3

Following an open inguinal hernia repair, a patient goes into acute urinary retention. You are asked to insert a suprapubic catheter (SPC) as urethral catheterisation has failed on multiple attempts. Which of the following is the correct landmark for inserting an SPC?

A) 2cm (2 fingerbreadth) below the umbilicus in the midline

B) 2cm (2 fingerbreadth) above the pubic symphysis in the midline

C) 2cm (2 fingerbreadth) above the pubic symphysis to the left of the midline

D) 2cm (2 fingerbreadth) above the midpoint of the left inguinal ligament

Question 4

When performing a scrotal exploration, identify the correct order of layers encountered from skin down to testis.

A) Skin, external spermatic fascia, internal spermatic fascia, dartos, cremasteric fascia, tunica vaginalis, tunica albuginea

B) Skin, cremasteric fascia, dartos, external spermatic fascia, internal spermatic fascia, tunica vaginalis, tunica albuginea

C) Skin, external spermatic fascia, cremasteric fascia, internal spermatic fascia, dartos, tunica vaginalis, tunica albuginea

D) Skin, dartos, external spermatic fascia, cremasteric fascia, internal spermatic fascia, tunica vaginalis, tunica albuginea

E) Skin, dartos, cremasteric fascia, external spermatic fascia, internal spermatic fascia, tunica vaginalis, tunica albuginea

Question 5

In the embryological development of the male genital system, testosterone release drives the second stage of testicular descent from the level of the inguinal ligament along the gubernaculum to the scrotum. What stimulates the first stage of testicular descent?

    A) Luteinising hormone

    B) Mullerian inhibitory substance

    C) SRY gene

    D) Follicle stimulating hormone

    E) Gonadotrophin releasing hormone

Question 6

You are asked to see a 3-year-old boy with a painful non-retractile foreskin. The parents are very worried that they are unable to retract the foreskin to wash beneath it and are asking for a circumcision. On examination foreskin is non-retractile, you are unable to see the glans and the child finds this painful and asks you to stop. There is no evidence of erythema or scarring to suggest balanitis xerotica obliterans. How will you proceed?

    A) Reassure and discharge the parents

    B) Perform a circumcision

    C) Perform a dorsal slit

    D) Prescribe a course of antibiotics

    E) Insert a catheter under GA

Question 7

A 1-year-old ex-prem boy is referred with concerns of an undescended testis. Since birth, the right testis has not been seen. On examination the left testis is within the left hemiscrotum and there is no testis visible in the right hemi-scrotum or groin. The testis is palpable in the groin and can be milked down to the scrotum. When released, it retracts back into the inguinal canal. What is the diagnosis and management?

    A) A retractile testis – keep under surveillance in clinic

    B) Undescended testis – keep under surveillance in clinic

    C) Undescended testis – plan for right-sided orchidopexy

    D) Undescended testis – plan for orchidopexy at the age of 2

    E) An ascending testis – plan for right orchidopexy

Question 8

A 4-year-old boy presents with a 24-hour history of a swollen right testis. On examination, he remains comfortable and there is significant swelling and erythema of the right hemiscrotum with erythema that crosses the midline. You are able to get above the swelling. What is the most likely diagnosis?

A) A delayed presentation of a testicular torsion

B) Torted hydatid of Morgagni

C) Epididimo-orchitis

D) Inguino-scrotal hernia

E) Idiopathic scrotal oedema

Question 9

A 16-year-old boy presents to A&E at 6pm having been kicked in the genital area 5 hours ago. You find a significantly swollen and bruised hemi-scrotum suggestive of a large scrotal haematoma. There is no ultrasound available at this time. What is your next step?

A) Admit for observation and organise an urgent ultrasound scan in the morning

B) Scrotal exploration

C) Organise a contrast CTAP

D) Urethral catheterisation

E) Attempt aspiration of haematoma to decompress swelling

Question 10

Below is an urographic phase of a an axial CT scan of a 23-year-old male involved in a blunt trauma to the back whilst playing football. What grade injury is this?

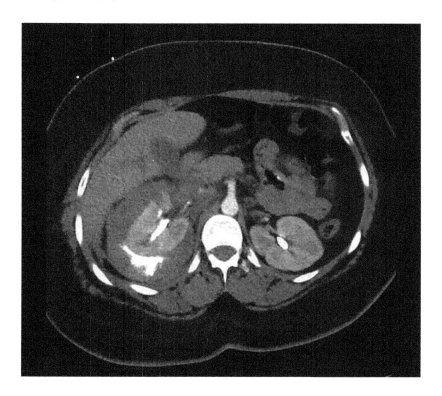

A) Grade 1

B) Grade 2

C) Grade 3

D) Grade 4

E) Grade 5

Question 11

The image below is of a patient who has been involved in a high-speed road traffic accident. They are stable in Resus in the emergency department with a pelvic binder on and an X-Fix is planned in theatre. You have been called as the patient has blood at the urethral meatus and the trauma team has performed a retrograde urethrogram. What would be the next most appropriate step?

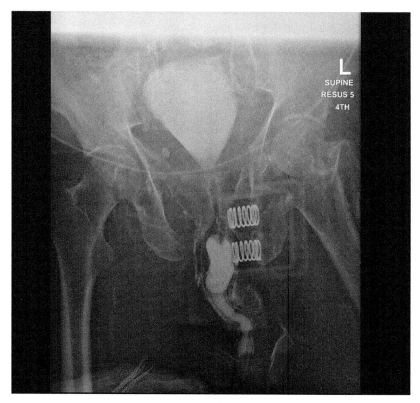

A) Gentle attempt at a urethral catheter

B) Supra-pubic catheter with a trocar technique

C) Radiologically guided SPC insertion

D) Take to theatre and perform and open cystotomy and SPC insertion

E) Bilateral nephrostomies

Question 12

This is an arterial phase CT trauma whole body of a 29-year-old male patient who was involved in a high-speed road traffic accident. What grade renal injury is shown?

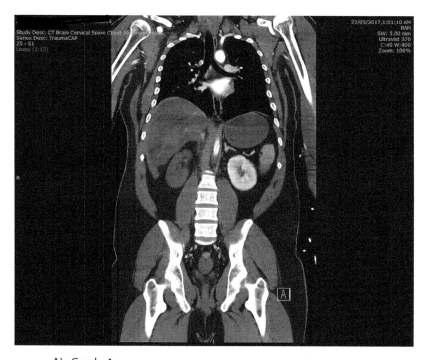

A) Grade 1
B) Grade 2
C) Grade 3
D) Grade 4
E) Grade 5

Question 13

This CT KUB coronal image is of a 49-year-old type 2 diabetic admitted with right-sided loin pain and a temperature of 38.5 degrees. She has been admitted by the surgical SHO and had blood and urine cultures taken. Her WCC is 17, CRP 136 and creatinine is 127. She is apixaban for a previous DVT. She has been started on gentamicin and amoxicillin as per protocol for urosepsis. The most appropriate next step would be:

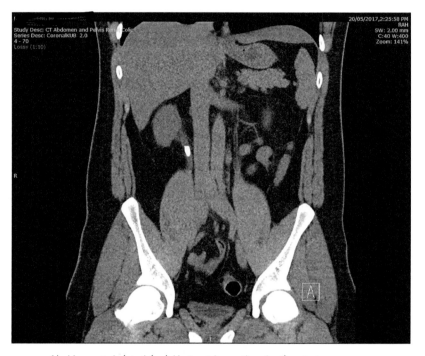

A) Urgent right-sided JJ stent insertion in theatre

B) Urgent right-sided nephrostomy

C) Urgent (in-patient) lithotripsy

D) Commencing tamsulosin 400 micrograms as a medical expulsive therapy

E) List for a primary right ureteroscopy on the emergency list

Question 14

A 16-year-old girl presents with bilateral loin pain and an USS confirms the presence of small bilateral stones. Her mother and older brother both suffer with recurrent urinary tract stones. What is the most likely composition of her stones?

A) Calcium oxalate

B) Calcium phosphate

C) Struvite

D) Cysteine

E) Uric acid

ANSWERS

CHAPTER 1 – LESIONS OF THE SKIN AND SUBCUTANEOUS TISSUE

Question 1a

Answer E – A rapidly enlarging ulcerated nodule on a sun-exposed site of an elderly patient should be managed with suspicion until proven otherwise.

Question 1b

Answer E – The most likely diagnosis from the appearance is squamous cell carcinoma. Radiotherapy would not give a tissue diagnosis. Curettage and cautery as well as shave excision would not allow the base of the tumour to be visualised and so should be avoided in suspicious lesions such as this. Given the likely diagnosis and high-risk features, excision with a 6mm margin is the most suitable option.

Question 2

Answer C – This painful nodule is in keeping with chondrodermatitis nodular helices, a common benign inflammatory condition of the ear. Patients often sleep on the affected side, and in this case the history of left hip and shoulder pains would be a triggering factor.

Question 3

Answer A – The stratum corneum is the outermost layer of the skin and provides mechanical protection from infection, dehydration, chemicals and mechanical stress. It consists of dead cells (corneocytes) surrounded by a lipid rich matrix (bricks and mortar).

Question 4

Answer D – Adenoma sebaceum are benign lesions found in tuberous sclerosis. They are commonly red flat lesions on the nasolabial folds and cheeks occurring in childhood. Bowen's disease is an SCC in situ of which HPV and solar damage are risk factors. Extramammary Paget's disease is a form of intra-epidermal adenocarcinoma. A cutaneous horn may have an underlying SCC so by definition is pre-malignant. Giant cell pigmented naevus are precursors of malignant melanoma.

Question 5

Answer D – This lesion is a basal cell carcinoma. All the options are reasonable except Hedgehog inhibitors, which are licensed for unresectable and metastatic basal cell carcinomas.

Question 6

Answer E – Although sun exposure is a major risk factor, up to 30% can arise in regions that are not sun exposed. The vast majority are nodular or nodulocystic and are more common in men.

Question 7

Answer E – High-risk lesions are those occurring in the immunosuppressed, recurrent lesions, lesions greater than 20mm and those on the eye, ear or nose. In addition, those with ill-defined lesions are also deemed high risk.

Question 8

Answer C – In a young, otherwise-healthy patient, the fibrosis and scarring from radiotherapy means that the alternatives are more preferable.

Question 9

Answer D – The latest consensus is that dermatologic procedures confer a lower risk for endocarditis. No prophylaxis is therefore indicated although individual cases should always be judged on their merits.

Question 10

Answer C – Clark's level and Breslow thickness relate to malignant melanoma. Bloom–Richardson grading relates to breast malignancy and the Fuhrman system relates to kidney cancer. Broder's grade of SCC consists of grades 1–4: 1) well differentiated, 2) moderately differentiated, 3) poorly differentiated and 4) anaplastic.

Question 11

Answer B – Guidelines produced by the British Association of Dermatologists advocate an excision margin of 4mm for lesions less than 2cm. This would be expected to remove the primary tumour mass in 95% of cases. For lesions greater than 2cm, a 6mm margin or Moh's microsurgery approach is recommended.

Question 12

Answer A – Studies have shown that a 3mm excision margin will clear the tumour in 85% of cases and a 4mm excision margin will achieve clearance in 95%.

Question 13

Answer D – In this case, a primary surgical excision would lead to a lower possibility of complete histological clearance. Moh's surgery is a technique whereby tumours are removed by staged excision and the surgical margins are examined completely. Indications for Moh's surgery include: BCCs of the central face, large or morphoeic BCCs, BCCs with poorly delineated clinical margins, recurrent or incompletely excised BCCs.

Question 14

Answer E – The majority of malignant melanomas occur de novo. The incidence is rising. Melanocytes are also found in the bowel mucosa and the retina. Superficial spreading malignant melanoma is the most common subtype. The risk factors for malignant melanoma are xeroderma pigmentosum, family history of malignant melanoma, previous melanoma, dysplastic naevi, red hair, immunosuppression and giant congenital pigmented naevus.

Question 15

Answer B – Breslow thickness is measured from the top of the stratum granulosum or the base of the ulcer, to the deepest point of tumour invasion.

Question 16

Answer C – Both BCC and SCC occur more commonly in immunocompromised renal transplant patients, but SCC is up to 100 times more common in contrast to the normal population.

Question 17

Answer A – Dermoid cysts are usually congenital and are especially located at the lateral aspect of the eyebrow. An underlying sinus may be present and will be palpable as a painless rubbery lesion that may contain unusual substances.

Question 18

Answer B – This is a pyogenic granuloma. Amelanotic melanoma is an important differential diagnosis but is unlikely given the short history and history of trauma.

Question 19

Answer E – Dermatofibromas are discrete solitary dermal nodules that arise following trauma or an insect bite. Pyogenic granuloma are benign haemangiomas that develop at the site of trauma. Histology is advocated to exclude the differential diagnosis of an amelanotic melanoma. Neuromas may occur spontaneously but are more common at sites of trauma or a surgical wound. Glomus tumours are derived from cells surrounding small arteriovenous shunts.

Question 20

a – O

b – J

c – N

d – B

e – D

f – F

g – G

h – K

i – I

j – L

CHAPTER 2 – ABDOMINAL WALL

Question 1

Answer C – Below the conjoint tendon lies no muscle but only fascia arising from transversus and the external oblique aponeurosis, and as such this is an area of weakness. The ilioinguinal nerve travels through the canal but lies outside the spermatic cord. The external oblique aponeurosis rolls at its lower edge to form the Poupart (Inguinal) ligament.

Question 2

Answer D – Although the risk of complications such as incarceration or obstruction is less than 1% each year, patients should be counselled to seek medical attention should this arise. Approximately one quarter of patients who initially opt for watchful waiting will require operative management for increasing symptoms.

Question 3

Answer A – A Kugel repair is a pre-peritoneal mesh repair. In the Lichtenstein repair, the mesh is sutured in front of the hernial defect. Mesh is not advised for paediatric hernia repairs and a herniotomy is usually sufficient.

Question 4

Answer B – This form of repair utilises the same plane as in laparoscopic TEP repairs. It is particularly useful in bilateral hernias or those with a large inguino-scrotal hernia.

Question 5

Answer B

Question 6

Answer E – Porosity induces tissue integration. Fibrosis due to mesh material yields a scar plate which will shrink in time. The minimum pore size should be 1mm but many meshes have pore sizes around 3–5mm.

Question 7

Answer B – The Lotheissen's approach is a trans-inguinal approach. The high approach allows pre-peritoneal dissection of the sac and facilitates the ability to assess and resect bowel if required. The low approach is generally used in the elective setting.

Question 8

Answer E – Treatment options include NSAIDS, anti-oestrogens, cytotoxic chemotherapy and surgery. Surgical excision is recommended as first line for abdominal wall and extra-abdominal desmoids.

Question 9

Answer B – This artery is often encountered when the hernia defect is extended medially.

Question 10

Answer E – If an umbilical hernia is still present by 3 years of age, operative repair is warranted.

Question 11

Answer C – Male gender is a risk factor for both direct and indirect hernia. Cystic fibrosis can cause chronic coughing. A low rather than high BMI is a risk factor for the development of a direct hernia.

Question 12

a – G
b – C
c – D
d – A
e – F
f – B
g – H
h – E

CHAPTER 3 – HAEMATOLOGY

Question 1

Answer E – Clotting screen was not required in this patient in first instance as there was no bleeding history and there were no haemostatic issues with previous procedures. Patient is not on anticoagulant either. Factor XII deficiency does not cause any bleeding complications and is of nuisance value in a routine APTT. Documentation is important so that in the future the patient does not face any problems related to a prolonged APTT.

Question 2

Answer B – As his creatinine clearance is reasonable, 2 half lives of Rivaroxaban is sufficient wait time to proceed to surgery and have adequate haemostasis. BCSH guidelines suggest that in case of low-bleeding-risk procedures and if CrCl>30ml/min Rivaroxaban can be stopped 24 hours pre procedure.

Question 3

Answer C – It is a standard advice to minimise risk of thrombosis, but only if haemostasis has been achieved and there are no bleeding complications post procedure.

Question 4

Answer E – As GCS is compromised, one cannot rule out a bleed and therefore one follows the principle of haemostatic correction/reversal first prior to further investigations as precious time can be lost and this will impact adversely on outcome.

Question 5

Answer D – This patient will require pre-operative factor correction and also repeated factor VIII concentrate infusions in the post-operative period until wound healing. The dose and interval will be determined by appropriate FVIII monitoring.

Question 6

Answer C – Rivaroxaban/Apixaban/Edoxaban are direct Xa inhibitors; Dabigatran is a direct thrombin inhibitor.

Question 7

Answer B – With cold agglutinin disease any surgery where blood will be cooled is a contraindication.

Question 8

Answer B – A platelet count of 50 is haemostatic for low-bleeding-risk procedures.

Question 9

Answer D – Prothrombin gene mutation is a low risk factor for venous thrombosis.

Question 10

Answer A – There is evolving evidence that direct oral anticoagulants should NOT be used in the antiphopsholipid syndrome due to lack of efficacy in this setting.

Question 11

Answer A – In view of no potential factors contributing to polycythaemia, primary bone marrow disorder (polycythaemia vera) is the most likely diagnosis.

Question 12

Answer B – This patient most likely has chronic lymphocytic leukaemia. Elevated bilirubin level gives high suspicion for autoimmune haemolytic anaemia, which is commonly associated with CLL. High MCV points towards large red blood cells which would be reticulocytes.

The diagrams below describe the metabolism of bilirubin.

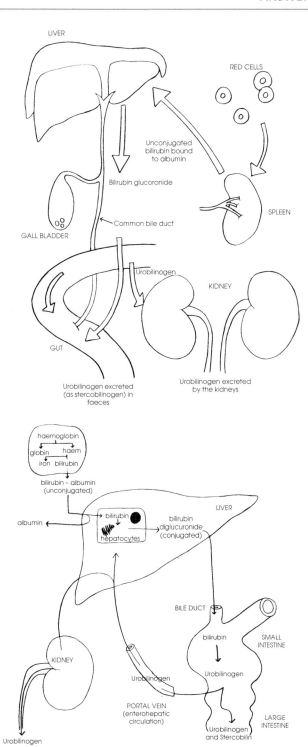

LIVER

RED CELLS

Unconjugated
bilirubin bound
to albumin

Bilirubin glucoronide

SPLEEN

GALL BLADDER

Common bile duct

Urobilinogen

KIDNEY

GUT

Urobilinogen excreted
(as stercobilinogen) in
faeces

Urobilinogen excreted
by the kidneys

haemoglobin

globin   haem

iron   bilirubin

bilirubin – albumin
(unconjugated)

LIVER

albumin

bilirubin

bilirubin
diglucuronide
(conjugated)

hepatocytes

BILE DUCT

bilirubin

SMALL
INTESTINE

KIDNEY

Urobilinogen

Urobilinogen

PORTAL VEIN
(enterohepatic
circulation)

LARGE
INTESTINE

Urobilinogen

Urobilinogen
and Stercobilin

Question 13

Answer D – Haemolysis screen that consists of direct antiglobulin test (DAT), bilirubin, LDH, reticulocytes, haptoglobin and blood film to look for spherocytes.

Question 14

Answer D – Splenomegaly is not usually seen in patients with myelodysplasia. All other disorders involve reticuloendothelial system and therefore splenomegaly is often seen, whereas myelodysplasia is a clonal disorder of haematopoietic stem cells characterised by progressive bone marrow failure.

Question 15

Answer C – Patients with Hodgkin lymphoma require irradiated blood products from the point of diagnosis for life. It is required due to defect of T-cell function.

Question 16

Answer D – Hodgkin lymphoma usually presents with painless rather than painful lymphadenopathy.

Question 17

Answer E – There is no evidence of any benefit of splenectomy in congenital TTP. In Evans syndrome (autoimmune disorder causing predominantly haemolytic anaemia and immune thrombocytopaenia), AIHA, hereditary spherocytosis splenectomy is used to stop auto-destruction of cells by autoimmune process and treat cytopaenias. In lymphoma, splenectomy may be performed for both diagnostic and therapeutic reasons.

Question 18

Answer B – The disease is localised only above diaphragm, does not involve spleen and there is no history of B symptoms.

Ann Arbor Staging Classification for Hodgkin lymphoma

Stage	Description
I	Involvement of a single lymphatic site (i.e. nodal region, Waldeyer's ring, thymus, or spleen) (I); or localised involvement of a single extralymphatic organ or site in the absence of any lymph node involvement (IE).
II	Involvement of two or more lymph node regions on the same side of the diaphragm (II); or localised involvement of a single extralymphatic organ or site in association with regional lymph node involvement with or without involvement of other lymph node regions on the same side of the diaphragm (IIE).
III	Involvement of lymph node regions on both sides of the diaphragm (III), which also may be accompanied by extralymphatic extension in association with adjacent lymph node involvement (IIIE) or by involvement of the spleen (IIIS) or both (IIIE,S).
IV	Diffuse or disseminated involvement of one or more extralymphatic organs, with or without associated lymph node involvement; or isolated extralymphatic organ involvement in the absence of adjacent regional lymph node involvement, but in conjunction with disease in distant site(s). Stage IV includes any involvement of the liver or bone marrow, lungs (other than by direct extension from another site) or cerebrospinal fluid.

Designations applicable to any stage	
A	No symptoms
B	Fever (temperature >38ºC), drenching night sweats, unexplained loss of >10% of body weight within the preceding 6 months
E	Involvement of a single extranodal site that is contiguous or proximal to the known nodal site
S	Splenic involvement

Question 19

Answer A – Transfusion related acute lung injury (TRALI) is caused by antibodies in the donor blood reacting with the patient's neutrophils, monocytes or pulmonary endothelium. Inflammatory cells are sequestered in the lungs causing leakage of plasma into alveolar spaces (non-cardiogenic pulmonary oedema). Most cases present within 2 hours of transfusion (maximum 6 hours) with severe breathlessness and cough productive of frothy pink sputum. It is often associated with hypotension, fever, rigors and transient peripheral blood neutropenia or monocytopenia. Chest x-ray shows bilateral nodular shadowing in the lung fields with normal heart size. (Handbook of Transfusion Medicine, editor Dr Derek Norfolk, 5th edition)

In the case above, TRALI is more likely than TACO due to:

- Young patient with no cardiac history
- Typical timing of symptoms
- Hypotension (TACO often presents with high blood pressure)
- Raised temperature (in TACO temperature is usually normal)
- Typical chest x-ray findings (in TACO, chest x-ray usually shows enlarged heart and typical characteristics of pulmonary oedema)

Question 20

Answer C – In βeta thalassaemia trait (heterozygosity) FBC usually shows normal or slightly reduced haemoglobin concentration, but low MCH and MCV. MCV <72 fl is usually strongly suggestive of thalassaemia. In the case above the level of anaemia is disproportional to the level of MCV and MCH, which hints towards βeta thalassaemia trait rather than iron deficiency anaemia.
The patient comes from Cyprus – there is a high prevalence of thalassaemia in Mediterranean area. βeta thalassaemia trait is usually completely asymptomatic condition.

Question 21

Answer D – HPLC (high-performance liquid chromatography) is now usually used as first line method to diagnose haemoglobin disorders. In βeta thalassaemia trait there is increased percentage of HbA2 haemoglobin (>3.5%).

Hb A consists of 2 α and 2 β globin chains
Hb A2 consists of 2 α and 2 δ globin chains
Hb F (fetal) consists of 2 α and 2 γ globin chains

Question 22

Answer B – Significant new thrombocytopenia in a surgical patient on unfractionated heparin warrants high suspicion for HIT. This patient has high HIT probability score and developed DVT so has Heparin Induced Thrombocytopenia with thrombosis. Management should include: immediate stopping heparin and starting alternative anticoagulation. HIT screen should be sent to confirm diagnosis; however, appropriate treatment should NOT be delayed whilst waiting for the results.

Thrombocytopenia
Score 2: Platelet Count decreased more than 50% from baseline with nadir >20,000
Score 1 Platelet Count decreased 30–50% from baseline with nadir 10–20,000
Score 0: Platelet Count decreased less than 30% from baseline with nadir <10,000

Timing after onset of current Heparin course
Score 2: Clear onset days 5–10 (or <1 day if prior exposure Heparin within last 30 days)
Score 1: Probable onset days 5–10 (or <1 day if prior exposure Heparin 30–100 days ago)
Score 0: Onset within 4 days and no prior Heparin exposure before this episode

Thrombosis
Score 2: Confirmed new clot, skin necrosis and systemic reaction
Score 1: Progressive, recurrent or suspected clot
Score 0: No thrombosis

Thrombocytopenia other causes
Score 2: No other alternative cause of Thrombocytopenia
Score 1: Possible alternative cause of Thrombocytopenia
Score 0: Definite alternative cause of Thrombocytopenia

Calculate cumulative score of all 4 components
Total Score 0–3: Low probability (less than 5% risk of Clinically Significant HIT)
Total Score 4–5: Intermediate probability
Total Score 6–8: High probability (>80% risk of Clinically Significant HIT)

Question 23

Answer A – It usually takes several weeks for neutropenia to resolve post viral infection. Causes of neutropenia include:

    a) Congenital e.g. Kostmann's syndrome

    b) Acquired:

       - Infection: viral infections, hepatitis, overwhelming sepsis
       - Drugs
       - Immune mediated: autoimmune neutropenia, SLE, Felty's syndrome
       - Bone marrow failure/infiltration: leukaemia, lymphoma, myelodysplastic syndromes, haematinic deficiency

CHAPTER 4 – GENETIC ASPECTS OF SURGICAL DISEASE

Question 1

Answer B – This pedigree demonstrates multiple affected generations with an average of 50% affected in subsequent generations. There is male-to-male transmission and males and females are equally affected. Therefore the most likely inheritance pattern is autosomal dominant.

Question 2

Answer D – The triad of hyperparathyroidism, phaeochromocytoma and medullary thyroid cancer is classic for multiple endocrine neoplasia type 2.

Question 3

Answer C – NICE guidelines recommend offering BRCA testing when the chance of identifying a mutation is 10%.

Question 4

Answer E – Breast cancer is common in the UK with 1 in 8 women being affected. The most likely reason for two post-menopausal breast cancers in a family is multifactorial inheritance, where multiple lower-risk genetic factors contribute to increased susceptibility alongside environmental factors. No genetic testing would be indicated in this family, but the patient would be deemed moderate risk and be referred for increased annual mammograms between 40 and 50 years, and thereafter 3 yearly through the NHS breast-screening programme.

Question 5

Answer B – Mutations in CDH1 cause hereditary diffuse gastric cancer.

Question 6

Answer C – In MEN2, thyroid cancer can occur below the age of 5. Depending on the exact mutation, genetic testing is recommended before age 5 so that prophylactic thyroidectomy can be performed in at-risk children. In MEN1, testing is recommended before puberty (between the ages of 10 and 13). The others are adult onset cancer syndromes and genetic testing in childhood is not recommended to enable the child to make an autonomous decision about timing of testing in adulthood.

Question 7

Answer C – Hepatoblastomas and young onset polyposis with a predominance of tubulovillous adenomas are associated with familial adenomatous polyposis (FAP). MUTYH polyposis is recessive and would not fit with the cancer diagnoses across two generations.

Question 8

Answer A – The only one of these patients who has a ≥10% chance of having a BRCA mutation is the 60 year old with high grade serous ovarian cancer. Patients with high grade serous ovarian cancer have a 10–20% chance of having a BRCA mutation regardless of family history. Mucinous ovarian cancer is not associated with BRCA mutations but can be associated with Lynch syndrome. The other women with breast cancer fall below the 10% likelihood of finding a mutation.

Question 9

Answer D – Von Hippel Lindau syndrome is associated with renal cell carcinoma, retinal angiomas, cerebellar and spinal haemangioblastomas, phaeochromocytoma and more rarely with pancreatic neuroendocrine tumours. However, the only patient who would get reflex genetic testing of the VHL gene here would be the patient with cerebellar haemangioblastoma, which is a rare tumour with a strong association with VHL. The patients with renal cell carcinoma, PNET and phaeo should be assessed to see if they have further personal or family history that may indicate genetic testing is necessary but in isolation would not require additional testing. Hyperparathyroidism is not associated with VHL.

Question 10

Answer B – Women with Lynch syndrome caused by MLH1 mutations have an increased risk of endometrial cancer and risk reducing hysterectomy alongside BSO should be considered from age 40.

Question 11

1)   A

Lynch syndrome is due to mutations in one of 4 mismatch repair genes (MLH1, MSH2, MSH6, PMS2). Tumour testing by either immunohistochemistry (IHC) for mismatch repair proteins or microsatellite instability testing will be abnormal in patients with Lynch Syndrome.

2)   G

Mutations in the CDH1 gene cause hereditary diffuse gastric cancer syndrome. Women with CDH1 mutations have an increased chance of developing lobular breast cancer.

3)   D

Cowden syndrome is caused by mutations in the PTEN gene and is associated with the development of harmatomatous bowel polyps as well as macrocephaly, autism and developmental delay and increased risk of breast, endometrial and thyroid cancers.

4) C

Peutz–Jeghers syndrome is due to mutations in the STK11 gene. Carriers develop histologically recognisable "Peutz–Jegher" bowel polyps, oromucosal hyperpigmentation and females have an increased risk of developing breast cancer.

5) H

PPAP syndromes are caused by mutations in POLD1/POLE and usually lead to hypermutated tumours which may have implications for oncological management with novel immunotherapies.

Question 12

1) A

Prophylactic daily low-dose aspirin has been shown to reduce bowel cancer risk in families where there is suspected increased genetic susceptibility due to polygenic or multifactorial risk factors.

2) D

Females with MSH6 mutations have an increased risk of developing both endometrial and ovarian cancer, as well as colorectal cancer. There may also be some risk reduction with daily low-dose aspirin, but risk-reducing gynaecological surgery of womb, fallopian tubes and ovaries would have the highest impact on future cancer risk.

3) G

Females with Cowden syndrome are at increased risk of thyroid, breast and endometrial cancer. At age 18 the highest immediate cancer risk is for thyroid cancer and risk-reducing thyroidectomy should be considered.

4) C

BRCA1 mutation carriers are at increased risk of developing ER – ve breast cancers. Tamoxifen is therefore not recommended as a risk-reduction strategy. Women may choose to start annual breast screening from age 30, with annual breast MRI age 30–40, annual breast MRI and mammogram between ages 40 and 50, and annual mammogram after age 50. Alternatively, they may wish to consider risk-reducing bilateral mastectomies. Ovarian cancer risk at age 31 would not warrant prophylactic bilateral salpingo-oophorectomy. This procedure would be offered from age 40 or after women have completed their families.

5)   F
Mutations in the APC gene cause familial adenomatous polyposis
(FAP). Depending on polyp burden, risk-reducing colectomy is often
necessary in the third decade.

Question 13

1 – B
2 – F (Lhermitte–Duclos disease)
3 – E
4 – G (Gorlin syndrome)
5 – D (hereditary paraganglioma-phaeochromocytoma syndrome)

CHAPTER 5 – ONCOLOGY FOR SURGEONS

Question 1

Answer C – Familial adenomatous polyposis coli is associated with
germline mutations in AP gene with an increased risk of papillary
thyroid cancer. Other inherited predispositions include Cowden
syndrome involving differentiated thyroid cancer, breast cancer and
multiple hamartomas.

Question 2

Answer E – The risk increases with an increased BMI in a dose-
response relationship.

Question 3

Answer D – Anthracyclines such as Doxorubicin are used in breast
cancer, bladder cancer and lymphomas. One of the most serious
side effects is cardiomyopathy and patients should have an echo
before treatment is started. The risk of anthracycline induced
cardiomyopathy is raised in those with hypertension, poor nutritional
status, older age and diabetes.

Question 4

Answer A – Imatinib has a role in the management of Gastrointestinal stomal tumours. Sunitinib acts on multiple target tyrosine kinase whereas imatinib acts on bcr-Abl.

Question 5

Answer B – Cyclophosphamide is an alkylating cytotoxic drug used both in malignancy and autoimmune diseases often in combination with other agents. Common side effects are leucopenia, hair loss, nausea and skin discolouration.

Question 6

Answer E – Capecitabine is used in breast, gastric and bowel cancer often in combination with another agent. It is rapidly converted to 5-FU in tumour tissue. Prior to each cycle full blood counts, renal and liver function tests are performed.

Question 7

Answer C – Trastuzumab is widely known as Herceptin and has a significant role in the management of HER 2 positive breast cancer.

Question 8

Answer C – In the UK the treatment duration is 1 year.

Question 9

Answer C – This factor limits the use of a CEA as a screening tool.

Question 10

Answer E

Question 11

Answer B – In 2006 the MAGIC trial looked at Perioperative FEC (ECF) vs surgery alone in 500 patients. 5FU + Epirubicin + Cisplatin. The regimen was 3 cycles of FEC followed by a 3–6 week break before surgery and then 3 more cycles of ECF after 6–12 weeks. The chemotherapy group increased 5 year survival 36% compared to 23% in the surgery alone group.

Question 12

Answer A – The FLOT trial looked at more than 700 patients given a regimen of 5FU+ Leucovorin + Oxaliplatin + Taxane- Docetaxel given pre- and post-op for resectable gastric or GOJ tumours. The treatment group had an increased progression free survival 30 months compared to 18 months in the standard group. The median survival and overall survival was 50 months compared to 35 months.

Question 13

Answer E – The TME dissection reduced local recurrence rates from 30% to under 5%.

Question 14

Answer B

Question 15

Answer D – Oxaplatin and 5-fluorouracil + folinic acid (FOLFOX) or 5-FU + folinic acid + irontecan (FOLFIRI) downsizes metastases allowing resection. A course of systemic chemotherapy is usually recommended to eradicate microscopic disease.

Question 16

Answer A – Recurrence following a resection previously is not necessarily a contraindication to a further resection and some units have published good results in appropriate patients.

Question 17

Answer E – Although HPV 16 and HPV 18 are implicated in the development of anal cancer, antiviral treatment is not part of the treatment regimen. External beam radiation and brachytherapy are used for local control. Anal SCC is a radiosensitive tumour.

Question 18

Answers:

1 – C	4 – B	7 – E
2 – M	5 – J	8 – G
3 – H	6 – D	

CHAPTER 6: PATHOPHYSIOLOGY OF SHOCK AND PERITONITIS

Question 1

Answer D – The European Society of Intensive Care Medicine recently (2016) redefined sepsis and its screening criteria. The original definition of SIRS, severe sepsis and septic shock is now defunct and replaced solely by:

Sepsis – a life threatening organ dysfunction due to dysregulated host response to infection

Hypotension: SBP less than or equal to 100 mmHg
Altered mental state: GCS <15
Tachypnoea: RR greater or equal to 22

Septic shock – a subset of sepsis in which cellular/metabolic abnormalities are profound enough to substantially increase mortality

Persistent hypotension requiring support to maintain MAP greater then 65mmHg
Lactate greater or equal to 2 mmol/L

Question 2

Answer C – Noradrenaline is an alpha receptor agonist and therefore will result in peripheral vasoconstriction. All the other answers, although improving cardiac contractility, would likely worsen the blood pressure.

Question 3

Answer E – Indications for renal replacement therapy:

Diuretic resistant pulmonary oedema
Refractory hyperkalaemia
Metabolic acidosis
Symptomatic uraemia
Overdose of dialyzable drugs

Question 4

Answer E – Alkalosis shifts the O2 curve to the left.

Question 5

Answer A – Overwhelming post-splenectomy infection syndrome is a rare but well-known complication of splenectomy, with the highest risk being splenectomy in children and haematological malignancy. It is characterised by a catastrophically rapid onset, massive bacteraemia and a high mortality rate. Post splenectomy patients are particularly susceptible to encapsulated organisms with pneumococcus accounting for 50–90% of all infections.

Question 6

Answer D – This lady has multiple risk factors for a DVT/pulmonary embolism and has symptoms in keeping with such. CTPA has the best diagnostic accuracy for a PE with a specificity of 96%.

Question 7

Answer A – ICP would increase due to a reduction in venous return from the cranium.

Question 8

Answer C – T10 marks the dermatome likely to be at the midpoint of the incision and therefore would give the most effective coverage of analgesia if placed here.

Question 9

Answer D – Although all these answers are respiratory complications of pancreatitis, the investigations are classic for the Berlin criteria for ARDS.

Question 10

Answer B – A typical male is composed of approximately 60% water. This is split into intra-cellular fluid, which is roughly 66% of TBW, and extracellular fluid, which is roughly 33% of TBW. Therefore, a typical 70kg male will contain approximately 42L of water of which 28L is in the intracellular compartment and 14L in the extracellular compartment. The extracellular compartment is further divided into interstitial fluid (75% of extracellular compartment) and intravascular fluid (25% of extracellular compartment).

0.9% Saline is isotonic and therefore will distribute within the extracellular compartment. 25% of extracellular compartment is intravascular; therefore 250mls will remain in intravascular compartment.

5% dextrose is hypotonic and will therefore distribute equally into all compartments. 66% of the dextrose will enter the intracellular compartment, leaving 333mls in extracellular compartment. 25% of extracellular compartment is intravascular; therefore only 84mls of 1L of 5% dextrose will remain in the intravascular space.

Question 11

Answer E – Left ventricular contractility is estimated from the gradient of the upstroke. Stroke volume is estimated from the area under the systolic portion of the waveform. Peripheral vascular resistance is reflected in the position of the diacrotic notch. Fluid responsiveness can be determined by changes in the 'swing' of the arterial line in response to changes in intrathoracic pressure with breathing.

Question 12

Answer A – All others exceed the toxic dose.

Max doses:
Bupivacaine = 2mg/kg
Lignocaine = 3mg/kg (with adrenaline 7mg/kg)
Ropivacaine = 3mg/kg
Prilocaine = 6mg/kg

Question 13

Answer D – Fat embolism typically presents as respiratory distress, neurological changes and petechial rash. Although the eyes can be effected (Purtscher's retinopathy), photophobia is an unlikely feature.

Question 14

Answer C

Question 15

Answer B – All patients under general anaesthetic are at risk of hypothermia as thermoregulation is lost. Outcomes are known to be worse following hypothermia. Patients are more likely to have bradycardia with hypothermia and this can progress to severe dysrhythmias.

Question 16

Answer A – Risk factors include:

Female
Smoker
Previous PONV
Hx of motion sickness
Use of opiates
Hypotension
Middle ear surgery
Ophthalmic surgery
Gynaecological surgery

Question 17

Answer C – Refeeding syndrome typically occurs within 72 hours of starting feed. It results from a sudden shift from fat to carbohydrate metabolism. A sudden rise in insulin leads to an increased cellular uptake of phosphate, potassium, magnesium and glucose leading to dangerously low serum levels.

Question 18

Answer C – 10mg oral morphine is equivalent to:

100mg codeine
60mg tramadol
5mg oxycodone

100mcg fentanyl is equivalent to 10m of IV morphine.

Question 19

1 – B
2 – G
3 – A
4 – C
5 – I
6 – H
7 – D
8 – E
9 – F

Question 20

1 – C
2 – F
3 – A
4 – D
5 – H
6 – I
7 – B
8 – J
9 – G
10 – E

Question 21

1 – D
2 – F
3 – I
4 – A
5 – B
6 – G
7 – H
8 – C
9 – E

CHAPTER 7 – SURGICAL NUTRITION

Question 1

Answer D – The ebb phase occurs prior to the flow phase. It is associated with increased sympathetic activity, reduced metabolic rate, decreased resting energy expenditure, increased gluconeogenesis and increased glycogenolysis.

Question 2

Answer B – The loss of nitrogen from skeletal muscle results in a negative resultant nitrogen balance.

Question 3

Answer E – In trauma there is a fall in glucose uptake by peripheral tissues. However, in sepsis there is an increase. The decreased peripheral uptake of triacylglycerols can lead to hypertriglyceridaemia.

Question 4

Answer D

Question 5

Answer A – The total daily energy expenditure consists of the resting metabolic expenditure, activity energy expenditure and diet induced energy expenditure. The activity energy expenditure depends on the type of physical work undertaken. 25–30 kcal/kg (105–125 kJ/g) are required daily.

Question 6

Answer E

Question 7

Answer B – Copper has a role in collagen synthesis; however, of those listed, zinc has the greatest role in wound healing. Studies have shown it contributes to membrane repair, coagulation, inflammation and immune defence, tissue re-epithelialization, angiogenesis and fibrosis/scar formation.

Question 8

Answer B – Although all the nutrients listed may have a degree of depletion in this scenario, the patient is likely to have Wernicke–Korsakoff syndrome as a consequence of thiamine deficiency.

Question 9

Answer A – Insulin stimulates the production of glycogen, fat and protein. This process requires phosphate, magnesium and thiamine. Insulin stimulates the absorption of potassium into the cells through the sodium–potassium ATPase transporter, which also transports glucose into the cells. Magnesium and phosphate are also taken up into the cells. Water follows by osmosis. These processes result in a decrease in the serum levels of phosphate, potassium and magnesium, all of which are already depleted.

Question 10

Answer C – Hyperglycaemia can occur in the context of excessive administration of glucose or inadequate insulin. Rebound hypoglycaemia occurs if the glucose is suddenly stopped. Hyperammonaemia rather than hypoammonaemia occurs in the context of L-arginine deficiency.

Question 11

Answer B – Disruption of the enterohepatic circulation of bile salts increases the incidence of gallstones. Gastric hypersecretion leads to peptic ulceration. Increased colonic absorption of oxalate leads to hyperoxaluria.

Question 12

1 – L
2 – L
3 – F
4 – E
5 – K
6 – O

CHAPTER 8 – ACUTE GYNAECOLOGICAL DISEASE

SBA
ECTOPIC PREGNANCY

Question 1

Answer E – Most ectopic pregnancies are thought to occur in the ampulla as this is the region of fertilisation – any tubal motility issues would prevent migration down the tube so implantation is most likely to occur at the site of fertilisation.

Question 2

Answer A – A major risk factor for ectopic pregnancy is the presence of tubal damage, which may be due to previous tubal surgery, pelvic infection or endometriosis. Smoking affects tubal function, so that eggs are less likely to be carried down through the tube into the uterus. In IVF, there is a risk of the embryo migrating into the tube if placed too high in the cavity.

Recurrent miscarriage is the recurrence of failed intrauterine pregnancies, usually in the first trimester, and is suggestive of normal tubal structure and function as these pregnancies have failed following successfully passing into the uterus.

Question 3

Answer B – Adnexal masses are seen in 50–60% of cases, an extrauterine gestational sac (either empty or containing yolk sac/embryonic pole) in 35–50%. In up to 20% of cases a small collection of fluid may be seen within the cavity: a "pseudosac". Free fluid is not diagnostic of ectopic pregnancy but is seen in up to 55% of ectopic pregnancies. It may signify rupture of the fallopian tube or blood leaking from the fimbrial end of the tube.

The double decidual sign, described as an intrauterine fluid collection surrounded by "two concentric echogenic rings", is seen in an early intrauterine pregnancy.

Question 4

Answer A – In women who have a history of fertility-reducing factors (contralateral tube damage including hydrosalpinx, previous PID, etc.) higher rates of subsequent intrauterine pregnancy are seen in those who have salpingotomy rather than salpingectomy. As such, tubal preservation should be attempted as first line. A laparoscopic approach is generally preferable to an open approach in most cases.

PID

Question 5

Answer E – The Rotterdam diagnostic criteria of PCOS requires the presence of 2/3 of the following: hyperandrogenism (clinical e.g. hirsutism or biochemical e.g. raised free androgen index), oligo/anovulation (leading to oligo/amenorrhea), the presence of multiple small follicles on USS seen in a "string of pearls" peripheral distribution on the ovary. None of these criteria cause pelvic pain, which is the major symptom of PID.

Question 6

Answer A – As per the 2018 BASHH guideline for the management of Pelvic Inflammatory Disease.

Question 7

Answer C – Laparoscopy may lead to early resolution of severe disease, but should only be considered if there has been no response to antibiotic therapy, a surgical emergency cannot be excluded, or in the presence of a tubo-ovarian abscess. Ultrasound guided aspiration of pelvic fluid collections may be equally effective and is less invasive. Although adhesiolysis may be performed in cases of perihepatitis, there is no evidence that this is more effective than antibiotic therapy alone.

Question 8

Answer D – Superficial dyspareunia is pain on attempted penetration. This may be due to lower genital infections (candida albicans, herpes simplex, trichomonas vaginalis), but is not caused by

PID. Other causes include size disparity (e.g. vaginal atrophy in post-menopausal women, and in those with dermatological conditions such as lichen sclerosus), vaginismus (spasm of pelvic-floor muscles causing temporary narrowing of the vagina) and psychosexual dysfunction.

Question 9

Answer E – PID usually results from ascending infection from the endocervix into the upper genital tract. Chlamydia trachomatis is the most common causative organism. Neisseria gonorrhoea, anaerobes and other vaginal commensals may also be causative. Pathogen negative PID is common.

ENDOMETRIOSIS AND PELVIC PAIN

Question 10

Answer D – Perihepatic adhesions (Fitz-Hugh–Curtis syndrome) are seen in PID. The other findings are all associated with endometriosis.

Question 11

Answer C – Radiological features of polycystic ovaries include the presence of multiple (>25) follicles in the ovary generally each measuring 2–9mm in diameter. Although they may cause ovarian enlargement, they do not cause pain.

Question 12

Answer C – Endometriomas are ovarian cysts containing a thick brown liquid substance within, whose appearance is likened to melted chocolate. This appearance is caused by old menstrual blood filling the cavity of the cyst.

OVARIAN MASSES, BENIGN AND MALIGNANT

Question 13

Answer D – Abnormal vaginal bleeding, or post-menopausal bleeding (as the majority of ovarian cancer is diagnosed in post-menopausal women), is a symptom associated with endometrial abnormalities (cancer or hyperplasia), as well as conditions of the cervix and vagina.

Question 14

Answer B – In pre-menopausal women under the age of 40 (especially in the first 2 decades of life), AFP, βhCG and LDH should be measured due to the possibility of germ cell tumours. Ca-125 in this age group is unreliable at differentiating benign from malignant ovarian masses due to decreased specificity. Other conditions which may raise Ca-125 include endometriosis and fibroids, as well as other pathologies causing peritoneal irritation.

Question 15

Answer B – Classically, ovarian or adnexal torsion presents with a sudden onset of severe pelvic pain associated with nausea and vomiting. Torsion occurs rarely, but is an emergency (especially in younger women) as the ovary +/- fallopian tube has twisted on its vascular supply, leading to ischaemia and infarction if left untreated. Of note, endometriomas are less likely to tort as they form adhesions to adjacent structures.

Question 16

Answer E – Simple ovarian cysts (thin-walled, unilocular, without internal structures) less than 50mm diameter usually resolve spontaneously in 2–3 menstrual cycles. These can therefore be treated conservatively and resolution checked by USS after a suitable period of time has passed.

Question 17

1 – E
2 – C
3 – B
4 – F
5 – G
6 – B
7 – D
8 – K

Question 18

    1 – H
    2 – C
    3 – B
    4 – I
    5 – J
    6 – E
    7 – A
    8 – D

Question 19

    1 – J
    2 – O
    3 – P
    4 – T
    5 – F
    6 – C
    7 – D
    8 – O

CHAPTER 9 – EVIDENCE-BASED MEDICINE AND STATISTICAL ANALYSIS

Question 1

Answer D – A research hypotheses is a clear, predictive and testable statement that relates to the outcomes of a specific experiment, either describing a relationship between the independent and dependent variables or the absence thereof. Hypotheses can be said to either 'directional' or 'non-directional'.

A directional hypothesis describes the nature of the predicted relationship between the independent and dependent variables, usually in positive or negative terms using quantitative indicators (e.g. more than, less than, increased or decreased). Sometimes, directional hypotheses predict the magnitude of this relationship (e.g. the incidence of epistaxis in patients on treatment dose enoxaparin will

be twice as great as in patients on prophylactic dose enoxaparin).
Directional hypotheses are usually constructed when the existing
evidence suggests which way the results of that experiment will go.

A 'non-directional' hypothesis only predicts whether a relationship
between the independent and dependent variables will or will not
exist and does not state the nature or magnitude of that relationship
(e.g. the incidence of epistaxis will differ between those patients on
treatment dose enoxaparin and those on a prophylactic dose).

Question 2

Answers: (i) b (ii) d (iii) e (iv) a (v) c

Question 3

Answer B – Any factor that can systematically affect the nature of the
findings of an experiment or undermine the objective interpretation
of those findings or effect a disproportionate attribution of
value or importance to them can be said to represent a source
of 'experimental bias'. Attribution bias describes a propensity to
inappropriately or unjustifiably 'attribute' an observed phenomenon
to a known variable within an experimental system or an existing
theory or explanation of an apparently similar phenomenon,
inferring a causal relationship in such a manner that does not truly
reflect reality.

Question 4

Answers: (i) e (ii) d (iii) c (iv) b (v) a

Question 5

Answers: (i) e (ii) c (iii) d (iv) a (v) b

Question 6

Answers: (i) e (ii) c (iii) a (iv) d (v) b

Question 7

Answer B – In order to be considered falsifiable, every research
hypothesis must be paired with an appropriately constructed
'null hypothesis', which is a statement that directly contradicts the

research hypothesis. However, it is important to remember that there are more ways in which a research hypothesis can be 'not-true' than simply being 'false'. A null hypothesis must, therefore, encompass all possible outcomes of an experiment whereby the research hypothesis is demonstrated to be 'not true' and must represent an absolute negative (or positive) reflection of the statement made within the research hypothesis.

Question 8

Answer C – The conduct of research, whether involving humans or animals or the inanimate, is guided by ethical codes of conduct that are akin to those by which clinical practice is likewise governed. As such, deception should be keenly avoided unless absolutely scientifically justifiable (i.e. where the study would be meaningless without it).

In this example, the surgical registrar is concerned that knowledge of her audit being undertaken would confound its results, through the action of demand characteristics. Demand characteristics describe a form of experimental bias whereby the behaviour of participants consciously or unconsciously changes as a result of either real or perceived 'cues'. Indeed, if members of the surgical department under scrutiny were made aware of the focus of the audit, they might increase their levels of compliance with the completion of weekend handover sheets for its duration.

Attempts to avoid the effects of demand characteristics can include concealment of the process of data collection or the nature of the independent and dependent variables or the research hypothesis, use of clear and specific instructions and the minimisation of contact between participants and the investigator.

Question 9

Answer B – Quantitative data is expressed in terms of numerical values denoting quantity, whereas qualitative data is expressed in terms of attributes or characteristics that cannot be expressed numerically, denoting quality or the 'meanings' that can be attributed to or derived from phenomena. A good qualitative study should be explicit (addressing a clearly defined clinical problem), systematic (using a fixed plan or method) and reproducible (the same outcomes can be obtained by someone else using the same approach). Qualitative data is non-standardised, unconfined and often dependent upon the subjective experience of both the researcher and the researched but can also be said to more faithfully reflect reality and provide a deeper and more nuanced understanding of the phenomenon being studied.

Question 10

Answers: (i) c (ii) d (iii) a (iv) c (v) b

Question 11

Answer D – A 95% confidence interval is a range of values that you can be 95% certain contains the true mean of the population. This is not the same as a range that contains 95% of the values. This range captures the uncertainty of the estimate. Larger sample sizes provide narrower confidence intervals as the greater the number of samples the greater the probability that the sample/estimated mean will reflect the true population mean.

Question 12

Answer D – The primary objective of a statistical analysis within clinical research is to infer the effectiveness of a treatment to a population of patients by exploring treatment response in a sample of representative patients. The P-value is a useful tool that can help a researcher understand the probability that an observed effect of treatment is the result of chance. A result is statistically significant when the P-value is less than the preset value of α. Conversely, a result is non-significant when the P-value is greater than the preset value of α.

In other words, the P-value can be said to simply represent the probability that, if the null hypothesis were true (i.e. there is no difference between treatment groups), the sample size used would result in a difference between groups with respect to the endpoint, as big or bigger than the one observed. This is why a P-value is often referred to as evidence against the null. The smaller the P-value, the more unlikely that the results would occur if the null hypothesis were true.

Question 13

Answer a

a = normal distribution

b = exponential distribution

c = skewed distribution

d = uniform distribution

The central tendency of normally distributed data is the mean value, which is represented by the centre of the curve on the x-axis. Normal distributions demonstrate a mean that is equivalent to the mode (the most common value on the x-axis) and the median (the middle value on the x-axis). Normal distributions are symmetrical, with half the data falling to the left of the mean and the other half to the right of the mean, on the x-axis. Standard deviation is a measure of variability and represents the typical distance, on the x-axis, of individual data points from the mean. Within a normal distribution, 99.7% of the data falls within 3 standard deviations of the mean, while 95% falls within 2 standard deviations and 68% within 1 standard deviation of the mean.

Question 14

Answer D – As the first nucleotide in the triplet may be any one of the four bases (A; C; G; T), the second may be any one of the four, and the third may be any one of the four, there are total of:

$$4×4×4 = 64 \text{ possible outcomes}$$

That is, there are 64 possible triplets:

(A,A,A); (A,A,C); (A,A,G); (A,A,T);
(A,C,A); (A,C,C); (A,C,G); (A,C,T);
(A,G,A); (A,G,C); (A,G,G); (A,G,T);

and so on.

Question 15

Answer B – As the first grade may be any one of the 3 outcomes (H; M; L) and the second outcome may be either one of two outcomes (P; N), there are total of 6 possible outcomes to both tests:

(H,P); (M,P); (L,P);
(H,N); (M,N); (L,N);

Question 16

Answers: (i) b (ii) e (iii) d (iv) a (v) c

A Summary of Common Statistical Tests

Type of Data	Test Name	Test Description
Categorical	Chi-square	Tests for the strength of the association between two *independent* categorical variables
	Fisher's Exact Test	Tests the association between two categorical variables when one has small numbers of patients in one or more of the crosses between variables (i.e. counts less than 5)
	McNemar's Test	Tests for the strength of the association between two *related* categorical variables (i.e. two repeated measurements from the same patient)
	Logistic Regression	Tests how change in the combination of one or more predictor variables predicts the level of change in a categorical outcome variable
Continuous	(Independent) T-Test	Tests for the difference in means between two *independent* variables
	Paired T-Test	Tests for the difference in means between two *related* variables.
	ANOVA	Tests the difference between group means when there are more than two groups under comparison
	Regression	Tests how change in the combination of one or more predictor variables predict the level of change in a continuous outcome variable
	Mann–Whitney U Test	Tests for the difference between two independent variables but does not rely on the assumption of normally distributed data
	Wilcoxon's Rank Test	Tests for the difference between two related variables (does not rely on the assumption of normally distributed data)
	Pearson Correlation	Tests for the strength of the association between two continuous variables
	Spearman Correlation	Tests for the strength of the association between two ordinal variables but does not rely on the assumption of normally distributed data

CHAPTER 10 – GI BLEEDING

Question 1

Answer D – The Glasgow-Blatchford score is recommended for pre-endoscopic risk stratification tool in upper GI bleeding. It encompasses more detail than the pre-endoscopy Rockall score including blood test results and presentation (i.e. presentation with melaena/syncope).

The Rockall score is less sensitive as a pre-endoscopy tool but is used to predict mortality and risk of rebleed post-endoscopy.

The AIMS65 score was developed in 2011 by Saltzman and colleagues, having collected data from >29,000 patients. Whilst some studies suggest it to be superior to the Glasgow-Blatchford score in predicting mortality, the Glasgow-Blatchford score is widely recognised to be the superior scoring system in predicting need for endoscopy.

The Forrest classification is a classification of peptic ulcer findings at endoscopy developed at the Royal Infirmary in Edinburgh by John Forrest and originally published in the Lancet in 1974. It was later validated by a group in 2013 that found it still has accurate predictive value for rebleeding. The risk of rebleed based on the Forrest classification determines the need for endoscopic therapy.

CLIF-SOFA score is used in the setting of acute on chronic liver failure and is not related to upper GI bleeding.

References

Acute upper gastrointestinal bleeding in over 16s: management. *NICE*. 2012. http://www.nice.org.uk/guidance/CG141.

De Groot, N.L., van Oijen, M.G., et al. Reassessment of the predictive value of the Forrest classification for peptic ulcer rebleeding and mortality: can classification be simplified? *Endoscopy*. 2014; 46(1): 46–52.

Forrest, J.A., Finlayson, N.D., Shearman, D.J. Endoscopy in gastrointestinal bleeding. *Lancet*. 1974; 2(7877): 394–7.

Saltzman, J.R., Tabak, Y.P., Hyett, B.H., et al. A simple risk score accurately predicts in-hospital mortality, length of stay and cost in acute upper GI bleeding. *Gastrointestinal Endoscopy*. 2011; 74: 1,215–24.

Stanley, A.J., Laine, L., Dalton, H.R., et al. Comparison of risk scoring systems for patients presenting with upper gastrointestinal bleeding: international multicentre prospective study. *BMJ*. 2017; 356:i6432.

Question 2

Answer C – The Rockall score was developed in 1996 by Tim Rockall and colleagues, who identified independent risk factors that were then shown to accurately predict mortality in GI bleeding. It includes clinical criteria as well as endoscopy findings with increasing mortality and rebleed risk with increasing score. 2 points are given if there is a history of cardiac failure/ischaemic heart disease or major comorbidity, but 3 points are given for renal failure, liver failure or disseminated malignancy.

Rockall Score

	0	1	2	3
Age	<60	60–79	≥80	
Shock	No shock SBP≥100mmHg, HR<100bpm	Tachycardia SBP≥100mmHg HR ≥100mmHg	Hypotension SBP <100mmHg	
Comorbidity	No major comorbidity		Cardiac failure IHD Major comorbidity	Renal failure Liver failure Disseminated malignany
Endoscopic diagnosis	Mallory–Weiss tear No lesion identified No stigmata of recent haemorrhage	All other diagnoses	Malignancy of upper GI tract	
Stigmata of recent haemorrhage at endoscopy	None or dark spot only		Blood in upper GI tract, adherent clot, visible or spurting vessel	

Rockall Score & Mortality/Rebleed Risk

Score	0	1	2	3	4	5	6	7	≥8
Rebleed risk (%)	4.9	3.4	5.3	11.2	14.1	24.1	32.9	43.8	41.8
Mortality risk (%)	0	0	0.2	2.9	5.3	10.8	17.3	27.0	41.1

References

Guideline 105: management of acute upper and lower gastrointestinal bleeding. *Scottish Intercollegiate Guidelines Network* (SIGN). 2008.

Rockall, T.A., Logan, R.F., Devlin, H.B., et al. Risk assessment after acute upper gastrointestinal haemorrhage. *Gut* 1996; 38(3): 316–21.

Question 3

Answer E – At the time of print (2018), there is currently no reversal agent for the direct factor-Xa inhibitors (e.g. apixaban, rivaroxaban) available in the UK. However, in the setting of acute life-threatening haemorrhage, most hospital protocols suggest use of prothrombin complex concentrate (e.g. beriplex) as well as fresh frozen plasma (FFP).

Andexxa® (Portola Pharmaceuticals, Inc., South San Francisco, US) the coagulation factor-Xa (recombinant), inactived-zhzo, has been approved for use in the US to reverse affects of rivaroxaban and apixaban.

Idarucizumab is licensed in the UK to reverse the effect of dabigatran (direct thrombin inhibitor) in event of serious/life-threatening bleeding. Haemodialysis can also be considered for rapid clearance of dabigatran.

For reversal of warfarin give vitamin K IV 10mg plus prothrombin complex concentrate/FFP.

References

Andexxa 2018 (prescribing information). South San Francisco, CA. *Portola Pharmaceuticals Inc.* Available at: http://www.andexxa.com/ [Accessed 24th December 2018].

Burnett, A., Siegal, D., and Crowther, M. Specific antidotes for bleeding associated with direct oral anticoagulants. *BMJ*. 2017; 357:j2216.

Siegal, D.M., Curnutte, J.T., Connolly, S.J., et al. Andexxa for the reversal of factor Xa inhibitor activity. *New England Journal of Medicine*. 2015; 373: 2,413–24.

Question 4

Answer C – The Forrest Classification for bleeding lesions within the upper GI tract was first developed by John Forrest at the Royal Infirmary in Edinburgh, published in the Lancet in 1974. It was later validated by a group in 2013, which found it still has accurate predictive value for rebleeding. Any lesions showing signs of active bleeding or signs of recent haemorrhage were shown to carry a higher risk of rebleed and therefore should have dual endoscopic therapy rather than medical therapy alone. This lesion has a visible vessel at the ulcer base and is therefore a Forrest IIa ulcer. The rebleed risk without treatment is 19.5%.

The Forrest Classification

Forrest Classification	Lesion Description	Risk of rebleeding (%)
Ia	Spurting haemorrhage	23.6
Ib	Oozing haemorrhage	19.0
IIa	Visible vessel	19.5
IIb	Adherent clot	17.0
IIc	Haematin on ulcer base	9.7
III	Clean based ulcer	1.1

Reference

Forrest, J.A., Finlayson, N.D., Shearman, D.J. *Lancet*. 1974; 7877: 394–7.

Question 5

Answer D

The Forrest Classification

Forrest Classification	Lesion Description	Risk of rebleeding (%)	Recommended Treatment
Ia	Spurting haemorrhage	23.6	Dual endoscopic therapy
Ib	Oozing haemorrhage	19.0	Dual endoscopic therapy
IIa	Visible vessel	19.5	Dual endoscopic therapy
IIb	Adherent clot	17.0	Dual endoscopic therapy
IIc	Haematin on ulcer base	9.7	Medical therapy alone
III	Clean based ulcer	1.1	Medical therapy alone

This lesion has a visible vessel at the ulcer base and is therefore a Forrest IIa ulcer. The rebleed risk without treatment is 19.5%. Any lesions showing signs of active bleeding or signs of recent haemorrhage (Forrest Ia-IIb) were shown to carry a higher risk of rebleed and therefore should have dual endoscopic therapy rather than medical therapy alone. Intravenous proton pump inhibitor is recommended as continuous infusion for 72 hours after endoscopic treatment for those lesions with high rebleed risk.

References

Grainek, I., Dumonceau, J., Kuipers, E., et al. Diagnosis and management of nonvariceal upper gastrointestinal haemorrhage: European Society of Gastrointestinal Endoscopy (ESGE) Guideline. *Endoscopy*. 2015; 47:1–46.

Heldwein, W., et al. Is the Forrest classification a useful tool for planning endoscopic therapy of bleeding peptic ulcers? *Endoscopy*. 1989; 21(6): 258–62.

Question 6

Answer D – The Rockall score is a post-endoscopic risk stratification tool to give accurate mortality and rebleed risk.

Rockall Score

	0	1	2	3
Age	<60	60–79	≥80	
Shock	No shock	Tachycardia	Hypotension	
	SBP≥100mmHg, HR<100bpm	SBP≥100mmHg HR ≥100mmHg	SBP <100mmHg	
Comorbidity	No major comorbidity		Cardiac failure IHD Major comorbidity	Renal failure Liver failure Disseminated malignany
Endoscopic diagnosis	Mallory–Weiss tear No lesion identified No stigmata of recent haemorrhage	All other diagnoses	Malignancy of upper GI tract	
Stigmata of recent haemorrhage at endoscopy	None or dark spot only		Blood in upper GI tract, adherent clot, visible or spurting vessel	

Rockall Score & Mortality/Rebleed Risk

Score	0	1	2	3	4	5	6	7	≥8
Rebleed risk (%)		4.9	3.4	5.3	11.2	14.1	24.1	32.9	43.8	41.8
Mortality risk (%)		0	0	0.2	2.9	5.3	10.8	17.3	27.0	41.1

Question 7

Answer D – The key features in this patient's presentation are the history of syncope and melaena. It can be helpful to confirm at presentation with digital rectal examination and postural blood pressure readings. Syncope gives a score of 2, whereas presence of melaena gives a score of 1.

Glasgow-Blatchford Score

Admission risk marker	Score component value
BLOOD UREA (mmol/dl)	
6.5–8.0	2
8.0–10.0	3
10.0–25.0	4
>25	6
HAEMOGLOBIN (g/dl) – MEN	
>13.0	0
12.0–12.9	1
10.0–11.9	3
10.0	6
HAEMOGLOBIN (g/dl) – WOMEN	
>12.0	0
10.0–11.9	1
<10.0	6
SYSTOLIC BLOOD PRESSURE (mmHg)	
≥110	0
100–109	1
90–99	2
<90	3
OTHER CRITERIA	
HR ≥100bpm	1
Presence of melaena	1
Presentation with syncope	2
Liver disease history	2
Cardiac failure present	2

References

Acute upper gastrointestinal bleeding in over 16s: management. *NICE* 2012. http://www.nice.org.uk/guidance/CG141.

Blatchford, O., Murray, W.R., Blatchford, M. A risk score to predict need for treatment for upper-gastrointestinal haemorrhage. *Lancet.* 2000; 356(9238): 1,318–21.

Question 8

Answer C – Whilst this patient obviously needs urgent endoscopy, this question is highlighting the importance of pre-endoscopy care. Resuscitation is key, but the intervention most likely to improve mortality in this patient group (variceal bleeds) is administration of broad-spectrum intravenous antibiotics to prevent against spontaneous bacterial peritonitis. Terlipressin, the vasopressin analogue, is indicated in suspected variceal bleeds with the aim of reduction in portal pressures.

References

Measuring the Units. A review of patients who died with alcohol-related liver disease. *NCEPOD*, 2013. http://www.ncepod.org.uk/2013report1/downloads/Measuring%20the%20Units_full%20report.pdf.

Tripathi, D., et al. UK guidelines on the management of variceal haemorrhage in cirrhotic patients. *Gut.* 2015; 0: 1–25.

Question 9

Answer E – This patient has uncontrolled variceal bleeding despite endoscopic therapy. Whilst balloon tamponade can be helpful, it is associated with significant complications and is only recommended as temporary salvage treatment whilst awaiting definitive treatment. The treatment of choice in uncontrolled variceal bleeding is transjugular intrahepatic portosystemic shunt insertion, which should be carried out in specialist centres once the patient has been resuscitated.

Reference

Tripathi, D., et al. UK guidelines on the management of variceal haemorrhage in cirrhotic patients. *Gut.* 2015; 0: 1–25.

Question 10

Answer D – Whilst the optimum timing of endoscopy will vary case by case, and certainly should be considered earlier in acute variceal bleeding, the British Society of Gastroenterology and NICE guidance is that endoscopy should take place within 24 hours.

References

Acute upper gastrointestinal bleeding in over 16s: management. *NICE*. 2012. http://www.nice.org.uk/guidance/CG141.

Siau, K., Chapman, W., Sharma, N., et al. Management of acute upper gastrointestinal bleeding: an update for the general physician. *Journal of the Royal College of Physicians Edinburgh*. 2017; 47: 218–30.

Question 11

Answer D – This lady has already had 2 attempts to control haemostasis endoscopically. The mortality risk from rebleed is significant and she therefore requires definitive treatment. Transcatheter arterial embolisation of the gastroduodenal artery would be a good option and would avoid general anaesthetic risk. However, that is not one of the possible answers and so the single best answer in this case is surgical intervention with laparoscopic repair and omental patch.

Question 12

Answer B – There are an estimated 140,000 Jehovah's Witnesses resident within the UK. For reasons of religious faith, they refuse allogenic blood transfusion and transfusion of primary components. However, a number of related treatments can be matters of personal decision and so it is important to discuss and document which treatments each patient would accept/refuse.

An Advance Decision can be made when a patient has capacity to make a decision regarding a treatment or situation that may later occur. It is legally binding if valid and shown to comply with the Mental Capacity Act. Advance Decisions should be treatment and situation specific and have to be signed by the patient and a witness. They are commonly used to document wishes to refuse certain life-sustaining treatments.

In this situation the patient has clearly stated that he would refuse red blood cells and has a valid Advance Decision to that affect. All patients in the UK with mental capacity have the legal and ethical right to refuse treatment. Therefore, it would be incorrect to transfuse the patient (A).

To stop all treatment would also be incorrect (C), as he has only refused certain treatments. As the team caring for the patient, all other options should be explored. The patient is compromised and the priority is to resuscitate whilst not breaching the patient's Advance Decision. Therefore, to wait for input from the medicolegal team would delay treatment.

Transfusion of intravenous fresh-frozen plasma may be helpful, but it is unclear whether the patient also refuses this blood product. IV crystalloid will be more helpful in acute resuscitation and treatment of the acute hypotension.

References

Caring for patients who refuse blood. RCS, 2016.

Good Surgical Practice. RCS, 2014.

Good Medical Practice. GMC, 2013.

Blood Transfusion [NG24]. NICE, 2015.

Consent: Supported Decision Making – a Guide to Good Practice. RCS, 2016.

Mental Capacity Act 2005.

Newcastle upon Tyne Hospitals FT vs LM [2014] EQHC 454 (COP).

Question 13

Answers: 1h, 2g, 3d, 4f, 5a

BSG and AUGIS (Association of Upper Gastrointestinal Surgeons of Great Britain and Ireland) guidelines recommend that if gastric or duodenal ulcers are identified at OGD, H.pylori should be tested and eradicated if positive.

There is no role for surveillance of duodenal ulcers. However, all gastric ulcers should be followed up with repeat endoscopy to ensure healing and exclude malignancy.

Oesophageal varices grade 2–3, or grade 1 with stimata of recent/ active bleeding should be banded at OGD. The patient should then enter a "variceal banding programme" and undergo repeat OGD+variceal banding every 2–4 weeks until the varices have been successfully eradicated. Non-selective beta blockade with agents such as propranolol or carvedilol are recommended as secondary prophylaxis of variceal haemorrhage in conjunction with variceal banding.

Failure to control active bleeding should warrant referral to specialist centre for consideration of definitive treatment with intervention such as transjugular intrahepatic portosystemic shunt. Sengstaken–Blakemore tube insertion is used as a temporary measure to stabilise the patient until definitive intervention can be performed.

Question 14

Answers: 1b, 2d, 3e, 4g, 5a, 6f

Mallory–Weiss tears often develop

The give-away drug history of naproxen use in question 2 should point towards a duodenal ulcer.

Haematochezia is rarely due to an upper GI bleed. This history is classic for inflammatory bowel disease, namely Crohn's disease, and the abdominal pain and recurrent bloody diarrhea would warrant further investigations including MRI enterography and ileocolonoscopy.

Coffee-ground vomiting is only positive for upper GI bleeding in 10% of cases. It would be reasonable to give the answer here as (e), but in fact the best match is answer (g). Many elderly inpatients develop oesophagitis. Risk factors include being nursed supine, medications such as aspirin, NSAIDs, tetracycline antibiotics, and nasogastric tube insertion.

The patient in scenario 5 is clearly unwell with evidence of hypovolaemic shock due to a variceal bleed. Chronic liver disease due to NAFLD is increasing in prevalence.

The patient in scenario 6 also has evidence of chronic liver disease but he is haemodynamically stable therefore it is less likely you would find an active variceal bleed at endoscopy. Chronic liver disease causing portal hypertension can also lead to portal hypertensive gastropathy with or without presence of varices. It is quite common for patients to 'ooze' from the mucosa due to concurrent coagulopathy and/or thrombocytopaenia. Treatment is focused on reducing portal pressures with non-selective beta blockade (e.g. propranolol or carvedilol)

Question 15

Answer D – The shock index is calculated by dividing the heart rate by the systolic blood pressure. If the shock index is >1, this is classified as an unstable GI bleed.

Question 16

Answer A – As per the aforementioned guidelines, every effort should be made to localise and treat the site of bleeding before surgery is considered. CT Angiogram has the advantage of speed of access and ability to assess the whole of the GI tract. It has high sensitivity and specificity but the patient needs to be actively bleeding at a rate of 1ml/min to be detected. If the CT identifies the source of bleeding, embolisation should be performed within 60 minutes.

Question 17

Answer E

Question 18

Answer B – The Oakland score comprises age, gender, previous LGI bleed, DRE findings, heart rate, blood pressure and haemoglobin level. Scores of 9 or more are classed as a major risk.

Question 19

Answer E

Question 20

Answer B – admission and colonoscopy on the next available list

Question 21

Answer B – The guidelines recommend that in those without cardiovascular disease a cut of Hb <70g/L is used to decide upon transfusion. One should aim for a post transfusion Hb of 70–90g/L. In those with cardiovascular disease a value of 80g/L is used as a cut off.

Question 22

Answer E – for stable bleeds both should be continued. For unstable bleeds continue just the aspirin. Dual antiplatelet therapy should then be restarted within 5 days of bleeding resolution.

Question 23

Answer D – Idarucizumab reverses dabigatran whilst PCC reverses the anticoagulant effect of rivaroxaban.

CHAPTER 11 – ABDOMINAL PAIN IN CHILDHOOD

ABDOMINAL PAIN IN CHILDHOOD

Question 1

a) 4
b) 5
c) 3
d) 8
e) 6

Question 2

Answer E – With the appropriate surgical experience (and appropriate surgical kit available), a laparoscopic approach can be used at any age.

INTUSSUSCEPTION

Question 3
Answer A – Peak incidence is in infants 5–7 months and 70% of patients are between 3 and 12 months.

Question 4
Answer D – In a clinically stable child a delayed repeat enema 30 mins to 2 hours later should be performed.

GROIN AND SCROTAL LUMPS

Question 5
a)   1 (idiopathic scrotal oedema)
b)   5 (hydrocele – after the age of 2 this is unlikely to close spontaneously)
c)   8 (testicular torsion)
d)   2 (varicocele)

ACUTE SCROTUM

Question 6
Answer C – The commonest cause of an acute scrotum in children is torsion of one of the testicular appendages (hydatid of Morgagni) – 60%.

PAEDIATRIC TRAUMA

Question 7
Answer C – the only correct answer. Trauma is the commonest cause of death in children over 1 year of age. An infant should have their head in the neutral position to maintain their airway. Hypotension is a late/preterminal sign in children and usually occurs when 30% of circulating volume has been lost. Isolated head injury is the most common finding in paediatric major trauma.

Question 8

Answer C – This is most likely to be a pancreatic injury secondary to an end on handlebar injury. In two-thirds of cases it is associated with a duodenal injury or other intra-abdominal injuries.

Question 9

Answer D – Although a splenic laceration can occur with a motor vehicle accident, it is not classically associated with the group of seat-belt injury pathologies

UMBILICAL HERNIAS

Question 10

Answer E – Some degree of umbilical herniation is present in almost 20% of new-born babies (more in premature infants) and because the anomaly occurs after involution of the umbilical cord, associated anomalies are rare. In the first 3–4 months of life, the bulge may increase a little before getting smaller. Almost certainly symptomless. Most umbilical hernias close spontaneously, common practice currently is to offer hernia repair to children just before they go to school to avoid issues of bullying – it is very safe to wait until this point to see if it closes without intervention because the complication rate is so low.

INGUINAL HERNIAS

Question 11

Answer D – Even if successfully reduced, a hernia should be repaired on the next available list

TONGUE TIE

Question 12

Answer D – In babies, most tongue ties are divided without any anaesthetic; older children will require a GA.

MECKEL'S DIVERTICULUM

Question 13

Answer D – Bleeding is typically painless but almost always settles spontaneously.

DUODENAL ATRESIA

Question 14

Answer B – Polyhydramnios is one of the diagnostic features antenatally.

PYLORIC STENOSIS

Question 15

Answer D – 20% family history rate; babies are typically hungry and ready to feed even after just vomiting; metabolic alkalosis frequently occurs; resuscitation and correction of electrolyte abnormalities must occur before surgery is considered.

Question 16

Answer D – All the above statements are true except D. The surgical treatment for a pyloric stenosis is a Ramstedt's pyloromyotomy – either open or laparoscopic.

CHAPTER 12 – UPPER GASTROINTESTINAL SURGERY

UGI SBAS AND EMQS

Question 1

Answer B – This patient has Barrett's oesophagus (gastric metaplasia replacing the squamous epithelium). A biopsy is needed to confirm the diagnosis. As per BSG guidelines, intestinal metaplasia is not necessary for the diagnosis but is so for surveillance of short (<3cm) segment Barrett's oesophagus. Although this is a premalignant condition, due to <1% conversion rate annually, the BSG guidelines have extended the surveillance period to be either 2, 3 or 5 years.

The Prague criteria allow uniform reporting of Barrett's in which both the circumferential and maximal margins are documented. This allows for comparison during surveillance.

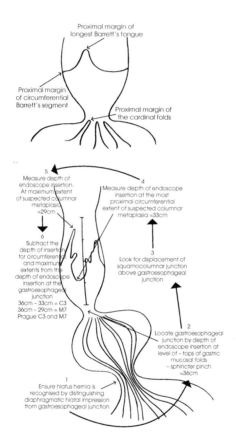

Question 2

Answers:

1 – f

2 – e

3 – a

4 – b

5 – d

6 – c
7 – g
8 – f
9 – j
10 – i

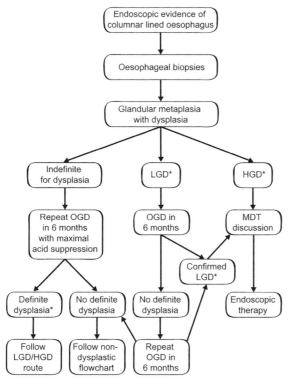

* dysplasia needs to be confirmed by 2 independent GI pathologists

Question 3

Answer C – Achalasia. This is a condition characterised by progressive loss of ganglion cells from myenteric plexus with hypertensive lower oesophageal sphincter (hence opens with a pop) and lack of oesophageal peristalsis. There is slight increase in risk of SCC. Biopsies are not needed for diagnosis. Antireflux procedure can be combined with Heller's cardiomyotomy but by itself will make the condition worse. Botox injection is reserved for unfit elderly patients. Cardiomyotomy and pneumatic dilatations are preferred options. Chicago classification shows 3 different types of the condition.

Question 4

Answer E – The stomach is a foregut structure entirely supplied by vessel of foregut viz coeliac artery via all 3 branches. The gastric tube blood supply is dependent on right gastroepiploic artery for Ivor Lewis oesophago-gastrectomy. The left gastric artery supplies lower oesophagus. Splenectomy may necessitate conversion to total gastrectomy due to concern regarding blood supply of the remaining stomach.

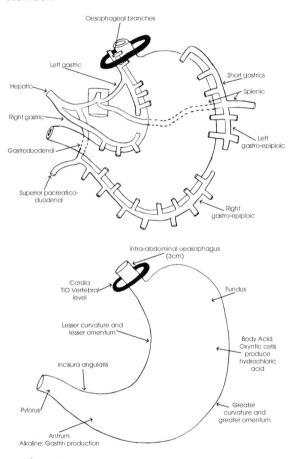

Question 5

Answer C – The right paracardiac (2), upper gastroepiploic (4sa), splenic hilum(10), distal splenic vessel (11d) lymph nodes need to be preserved and can only be removed if the patient is having total gastrectomy and splenectomy.

Question 6

Answer D – Staging laparoscopy will not influence treatment options in this case. It is used in patients with lower oesophageal, junctional and gastric cancers and can alter treatment in up to 30% cases.

Question 7

Answer C

Siewert classification of GE junctional adeno carcinoma

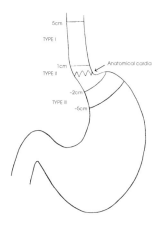

Question 8

Answer D – A 6cm GIST has intermediate/high risk of malignant potentials hence best course of action will be surgical excision. As the tumour is on the fundus, best treatment will be stomach conserving wedge resection with adequate margins. Lymph nodes are not removed due to low risk of involvement. Primary imatinib is given for inoperable and large GIST to shrink size.

Risk	Tumor size	Mitotic count
Very low risk	<2 cm	<5/50 HPF
Low risk	2–5 cm	<5/50 HPF
Intermediate risk	<5 cm	6–10/50 HPF
	5–10 cm	<5/50 HPF
High risk	>5 cm	>5/50 HPF
	>10 cm	Any mitotic rate
	Any size	>10/50 HPF

Question 9

Answer E – All are indications for endoscopic removal of the foreign body.

Question 10

Answer C – Unwell patients over 70 tolerate laparoscopic surgery poorly and hence should have open approach. Half of the perforated peptic ulcers have sealed spontaneously at the time of admission. Nevertheless, non-operative treatment can lead to collections and sepsis. Hence surgery after resuscitation is preferred. Older patients above 70 are poor responders to conservative management and hence this should be reserved for high-risk category patients and those who decline surgery. In such cases a CT guided drainage of collection can be useful. Elderly patients are better off having open surgery as against laparoscopic although latter should be a preferred method in younger patients with multiple benefits, such as less need for analgesia, shorter hospital stay, less wound infection and lower mortality.

Question 11

Answers A and B – Both are correct statements. Meckler's triad (vomiting, chest pain and subcutaneous emphysema), although diagnostic, is seen in only 15% patients. The single long oesophageal perforation is in left lower posterolateral position. Conservative treatment usually is unsuccessful due to significant mediastinal and pleural cavity contamination.

Question 12

Answer C – The Demeester score consists of 6 factors as below (with normal values in brackets):

Supine reflux @pH <4 (3%)
Upright reflux @pH <4 (8%)
Total reflux @pH <4 (5%)
Number of episodes (50)
Number of episodes lasting >5 minutes (3)
Longest episode in minutes (20)

Although symptom index (50%) is not part of Demeester score, it is calculated along with the symptom association probability (>95%) and both are taken into consideration when offering surgery.

Question 13

Answer B – The patient should have an immediate OGD in theatre to rule out gastric ischaemia and for NG tube insertion. The aspiration of the gastric content in such cases can cause spontaneous reduction of the volvulus. If the stomach wall is ischaemic already, then surgery is needed. Blind insertion of NG tube can cause perforation or aspiration. Conservative management and delayed OGD can lead to deterioration in patient condition.

Question 14

Answer E – The remaining indications are persistent vomiting and progressive unintentional weight loss. The obstructive jaundice should prompt urgent referral for radiological investigations.

Question 15

Answer B – It's recommended to take the patient for second OGD and attempt to stop bleeding, failing which interventional radiology is next option provided the patient is stable. Unstable patients need urgent surgery but an OGD may be attempted on the operating table first. The tranexamic acid is found useful in trauma cases (CRASH2 trial) but not in upper GI bleeding cases (meta-analysis by Gludd et al. 2012).

Question 16

Answer C – It is important to assess the oesophageal damage and degree of burns at earliest opportunity while protecting the airway in these cases. The patients with impending airway obstruction may need intubation straight away in A/E. Blind NG tube insertion can be dangerous. The antidotes release more heat and cause further damage and hence should be avoided. Contrast swallow examination is not indicated in acute situation.

Question 17

Answer A – The intra-abdominal pressure is positive at 5 mm Hg and creates a gradient of about 10 mm Hg as against the negative 5 mm Hg intrathoracic pressure thus preventing acid reflux.

The following are all factors that assist in preventing gastro-oesophageal reflux.

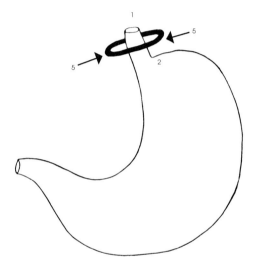

1. Cura. Mostly right but together giving effectively a circle of muscle.

2. Angle of oesophagogastric junction.

3. Apposition of mucosal folds.

4. Phrenico – Oesophageal ligament (a fold of connective tissue).

5. Intra-abdominal pressure acting laterally on small section of intra-abdominal oesophagus.

6. High pressure zone in LOS.

Question 18

Answer D – Endoluminal USS is done to assess the tumour and lymph nodes and to take samples from lymph nodes.

Question 19

Answer D – This is early cancer and hence patient can proceed to surgery without need for neoadjuvant chemotherapy. The radical chemo-radiotherapy is used for squamous cell carcinoma. The T2 tumours are not considered for endoscopic treatment as muscle layer is already involved. The staging laparoscopy has no role in tumours of mid oesophagus.

Question 20

Answers:

1 – G
2 – C
3 – A
4 – H
5 – I
6 – D
7 – E
8 – F
9 – J
10 – B

Question 21

Answer D – Peptic ulcers are the most common cause of UGI bleeding, accounting for 36% cases. Varices account only for 11%. Oesophagitis accounts for 24% of cases and gastritis + erosion for 22%. Mallory–Weiss tears and malignancy are responsible for around 4% cases each (Hearnshaw et al., GUT, 2011 – a UK audit 2007).

Historical operations for peptic ulcer disease included Billroth I (gastroduodenal anastomosis) and Billroth II (gastrojejunal anastomosis).

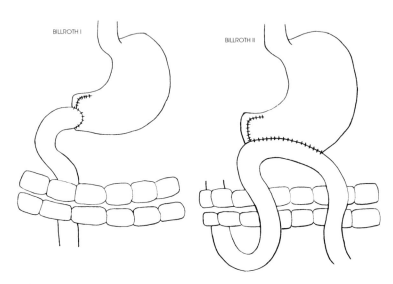

Question 22

Answer A – Although age forms part of the Rockall scoring system, it's divided into the three age groups <60, 60–79 and >80.

Rockall Scoring System				
Variable	Score=0	Score =1	Score =2	Score =3
Age (years)	<60	60-79	>80	
Comorbidity			Congestive heart failure, ischemic heart disease	Renal failure, liver disease, metastatic disease
Shock	No shock	Pulse > 100 bpm	Systolic BP <100 mmHg	
Source of bleeding	Mallory-Weiss Tear	All other diagnoses: e.g., esophagitis, gastritis, peptic ulcer disease, varices	Malignancy	
Stigmata of recent bleeding	None		Adherent clot or spurting vessel	

Question 23

Answer C – Stricture is usually a delayed complication and presents with difficulty swallowing. All the other complications can be responsible for the patient's symptoms.

Question 24

Answer A – In the West, the gastric cancer has migrated proximally in recent years where as in Asia it's mainly a disease of the distal stomach.

Question 25

Answer E

Question 26

Answer A – Bleeding is the most common presentation amounting to 50% of cases, followed by pain 20–50% and obstruction 10–30%. Asymptomatic cases are 20%. Weight loss is not a recognised presenting symptom for GIST.

Question 27

Answer C – This test is done for insulinoma. All other tests are done for gastrinoma.

Question 28

Answer B – It is indicated for staging of ca oesophagus only if the CT scan suggests lymph nodes involvement and is not of any value in early cancers.

Question 29

Answer A – Antireflux surgery is indicated for patients who don't wish to take long-term medications. The open surgery is not done anymore due to benefits of laparoscopic procedures. The gastropexy is not indicated for sliding type of hiatus hernia. The LINX procedure has not received widespread acceptance as a routine antireflux procedure as yet.

Question 30

Answer E – The transection is an historic method not practised any more.

Question 31

Answer C – The condition can be initially treated conservatively for smaller leaks. Prompt surgery is indicated for major leaks. Surgery is also undertaken for those leaks that fail to seal.

Question 32

Answers A and B – Both appear reasonable first steps and hence either of the answers should be correct. A quick X-ray in a stable patient can help diagnose a slipped gastric band; however, as this patient has had a gastric band adjustment recently and you are suspecting a tight band, first emptying the balloon appears to be a more logical answer.

Question 33

Answer D – The NICE guidelines state that the BMI limit is brought down in this group by 2.5.

CHAPTER 13 – HPB SURGERY

Question 1

Answer B – Whilst an ultrasound would be useful in identifying biliary duct dilatation, in view of the patient's age, presentation of painless jaundice and in particular weight loss malignancy would need to be excluded and therefore a CT would be more beneficial.

Question 2

Answer A – The blood profile in this picture suggests a possible hepatic picture and although it would be prudent to investigate with a hepatitis screen, an ultrasound would also be required to exclude choledocholithiasis.

Question 3

Answer C – An obstructive liver function picture with a dilated common bile duct is an indication for an MRCP. The lack of visualisation of the distal bile duct further strengthens the case. Although the patient may require a subsequent ERCP, the risks posed by the invasive procedure would require confirmation of pathology of choledocholiathiasis or pancreatic pathology.

Question 4

Answer E – The common bile duct can dilate post cholecystectomy. However, an MRCP would still be required to exclude retained stones given the presentation.

Question 5

Answer A

Question 6

Answer E

Question 7

Answer A – Given the presence of liver metastases, it is unlikely the patient will come to surgery. The next step would be to achieve biliary decompression and obtain cytology. In this scenario a metal stent would be preferable to a plastic stent.

Question 8

Answer A – Meta-analysis data has shown that pre-procedure diclofenac or indomethacin reduces the incidence of post ERCP induced pancreatitis.

Question 9

Answer A – The ideal management for biliary colic would be a laparoscopic cholecystectomy.

Question 10

Answer B

Question 11

Answer C – As the patient is elderly, frail and co-morbid the stress of surgery may be too much and thus initial focus should be to drain the sepsis in the form of a cholecystostomy.

Question 12

Answer D – The patient has cholangitis and his sepsis should improve following stone extraction at ERCP. Operative management at this stage would be reserved for failed endoscopic treatment.

Question 13

Answer B

Question 14

Answer C – The splenic vein joins the inferior mesenteric vein that joins superior mesenteric vein to form portal vein at back of neck of pancreas.

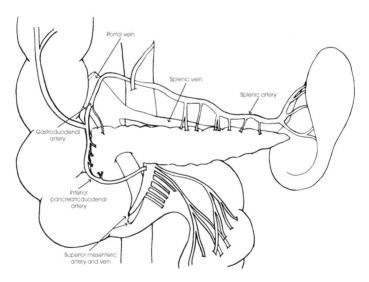

Question 15

Answer E – In ITP the spleen is usually of normal size.

Causes of splenomegaly – CHINA

Congestion: portal vein thrombosis, splenic vein thrombosis
Cysts: congenital – simple, dermoid, haemangioma
acquired – trauma, pseudocyst
Haematological: sickle cell, hereditary spherocytosis, thalassemia, haemolytic anaemias,
Infection: abscess, TB, schistosomiasis, malaria, EBV, CMV, HIV, typhoid, hydatid
Neoplasms: CML, lymphoma, myelofibrosis
Autoimmune: rheumatoid arthritis, SLE, sarcoidosis

Question 16

Answer D – The usual organism is echinococcus granulosus, which is commonly found in dogs and sheep. The majority of cysts are in the right liver lobe (70%), 15% left, 15% bilateral. However, they are also seen in the spleen, lung, bones and brain.

Diagnosis: incidental, CXR, USS, CT, MRI; ELISA or indirect hemagglutation test (IHA); eosinophilia

Gharbi's classification: Type I – cystic fluid; Type II – membrane separation; Type III – septa; Type IV – heterogenous; Type V – completely calcified

Treatment: albendazole/mebendazole 400 BD x28 days (3 cycles with 2 weeks gaps)

PAIR protocol: risk anaphylaxis, sclerosing cholangitis; Puncture, Aspirate – if no bile – Inject (ethanol 95%), Reaspirate x 3 times

Surgery: albendazole x 28 days; open surgery; hypertonic saline packs, intraop USS to locate; anaesthetist ready with adrenaline (anaphalyxis); PAIR done introperatively x 3ce. The liver resected with intact cyst with liver margin (Badria). This is useful for peripheral lesions. For intralobar lesions, endocyst is peeled out after decompression with PAIR protocol. Cavity can be marsupialised or filled with omentum or plicated.

Question 17

Answer E

Csendes classification I–V

I   Extrinsic compression of CHD by stones in cystic duct or Hartman's pouch

II   Cholecystobiliary fistula involving less than 1/3 of the circumference of the bile duct

III Cholecystobiliary fistula involving 1/3–2/3 of the circumference of the bile duct.

IV   Cholecystobiliary fistula with complete obstruction of the bile duct

V   One of the above + cholecysto- duodenal or colonic fistula

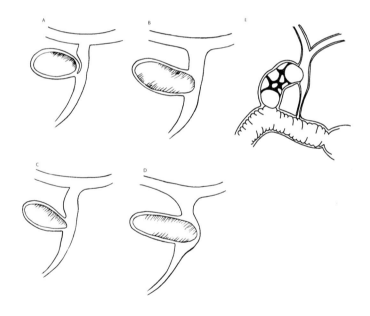

Question 18

Answer A – Choledochal cysts usually present in childhood.

There is a 12% risk of adenocarcinoma, which is why they require cyst excision. Liver resection is usually reserved for types 4 and 5. Types 1-3 are treated with excision of cyst and Roux en Y Hepatico-jejunostomy.

The Kasai operation is used in biliary atresia amongst infants.

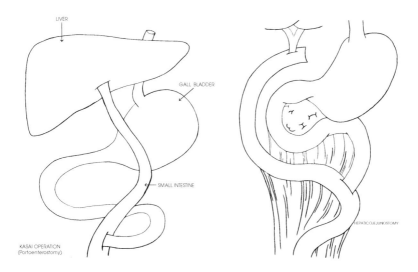

Todani Classification

I   Most common 70–80% fusiform dilatation of CBD; Ia cystic Ib fusiform; treatment – hepatico-jejunostomy

II   Diverticulum of CBD 2%; treatment – excision of the cyst

III   Choledochocoeles – diverticulum within pancreas or intraduodenal <1.5%; treatment – transduodenal excision of the cyst

IV   2nd most common 20%; intra and extrahepatic multiple cysts including choledochocoele; treatment – hepatico-jejunostomy + segment IV excision; IVa – intra + extra hepatic ducts multiple cysts; IVb – multiple extra hepatic cysts only

V   Caroli's disease; intrahepatic cystic disease with no choledochal cysts; segmental (hepatectomy) or diffuse (stenting, drainage, antibiotics, transplant); 10%

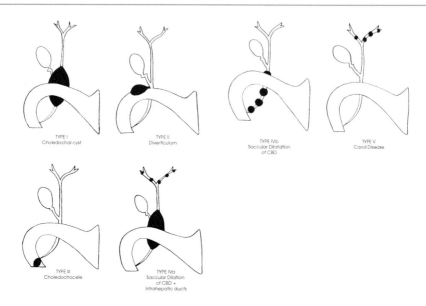

TYPE I
Choledochal cyst

TYPE II
Diverticulum

TYPE IVb
Saccular Dilatation
of CBD

TYPE V
Caroli Disease

TYPE III
Choledochocele

TYPE IVa
Saccular Dilation
of CBD +
Intrahepatic ducts

Question 19
Answer D

Question 20
Answer A – The Strasberg classification

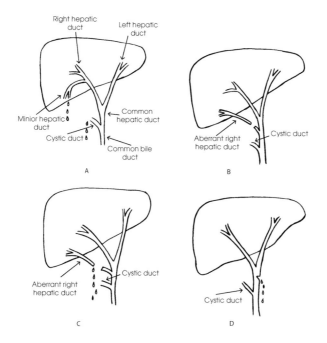

Right hepatic
duct

Left hepatic
duct

Minior hepatic
duct

Cystic duct

Common
hepatic duct

Common bile
duct

A

Aberrant right
hepatic duct

Cystic duct

B

Aberrant right
hepatic duct

Cystic duct

C

Cystic duct

D

Question 21

Answer A – Also called peri-hilar cholangiocarcinoma

The Bismuth–Corlette Classification

This is a classification for perihilar cholangiocarcinoma based on the degree of ductal infiltration.

> Type I – limited to the common hepatic duct below the confluence of the right and left hepatic ducts
>
> Type II – Involves the confluence of the right and left hepatic ducts
>
> Type IIIa – Type II and extends to the bifurcation of the right hepatic duct
>
> Type IIIb – Type II and extends to the bifurcation of the left hepatic duct
>
> Type IV – Extends to the bifurcation of both left and right hepatic ducts or multifocal involvement

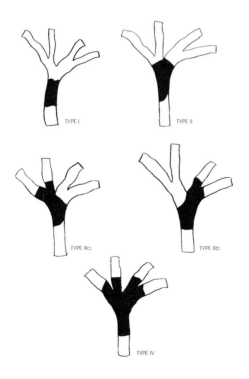

Question 22

Answer E – The gastroduodenal and splenic arteries arise from the coeliac artery. The superior pancreaticoduodenal artery arises from the gastroduodenal.

Question 23

Answer B – The Atlanta classification (2012) requires 2 out of the following 3 characteristics to make a diagnosis of pancreatitis:

1. Amylase x 3 times upper normal limit or lipase x 3 times upper normal limit
2. Characteristic imaging findings on CT/MRI
3. Epigastric pain

Question 24

Answer B – A white cell count more than 15mmol/L is part of the criteria. A score of 3 or more within the first 48 hours signifies severe pancreatitis.

Question 25

Answer A – Of the factors stated, only early enteral feeding has been shown to have proven outcome benefit in pancreatitis.

Question 26

Answer E – Risk factors include: smoking, chronic pancreatitis (alcohol), hereditary pancreatitis, blood group A, BRAC1, high-fat diet, Lynch syndrome, Peutz–Jegher syndrome FAP, MEN1, 2 relatives with pancreatic cancer, diabetes, obesity and alcohol abuse

Question 27

Answer D – Ductal adenocarcinomas comprise 85% of pancreatic cancers.

Question 28

Answer C

Whipple's Pancreaticoduodenectomy with the pancreatico-jejunal anastomosis, choledocho-jejunostomy and gastrojejunostomy

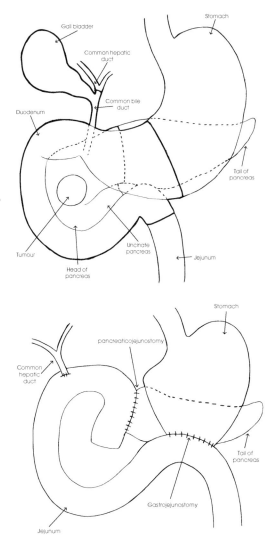

Question 29

Answer C

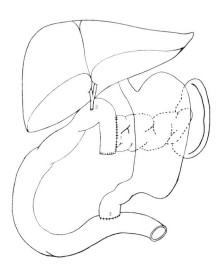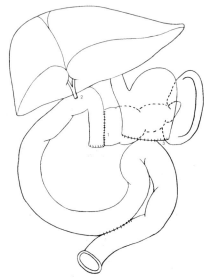

Pylorus preserving pancreatico duodenectomy	Whipple's pancreatico duodenectomy
Pancreatico-jenunostomy	Pancreatico-jejunal anastomosis
Choledocho-jenunostomy	Choledocho-jejunostomy
Duodeno-jejunostomy	Gastrojejunostomy

Question 30

Answer C – Both serous cystadenoma and single side branch IPMN have a low risk for malignant potential.

The following diagrams depict the morphological classification of IPMN. Main branch IPMN has a 50% malignant potential, in comparison to side branch IPMN 10% and MCN 17%. Assuming fitness for surgery, those with main branch IPMN should undergo resection. Those with branch duct IPMN if symptomatic, greater than 3cm or a CA19-9 greater than 25 should also undergo resection.

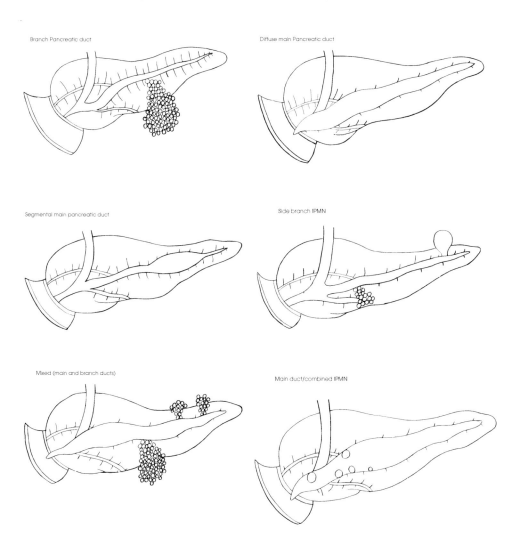

Branch Pancreatic duct

Diffuse main Pancreatic duct

Segmental main pancreatic duct

Side branch IPMN

Mixed (main and branch ducts)

Main duct/combined IPMN

Question 31

Answer B

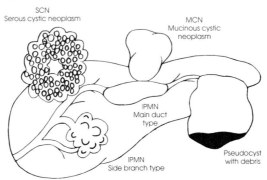

Question 32

Answer A – 85% of pancreatic neuroendocrine tumours are non-functional.

Question 33

Answer D – In contrast to a normal physiological state, gastrin levels rise rather than fall following exogenous secretin. This is the basis of the secretin suppression test.

90% of Gastrinomas are found within the Gastrinoma triangle / Passaro's triangle. This has borders superiorly of the junction of the cystic duct and common bile duct, medially the neck and body of the pancreas and inferiorly the D2/D3 junction.

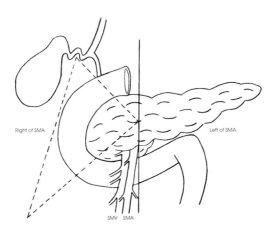

Question 34

Answer D – They arise from the alpha cells of the pancreas. 90% are malignant and therefore somatostatin analogues and surgical resection form the mainstay of treatment. Weight loss and glucagon levels >1,000 are a feature.

Question 35
Answer B

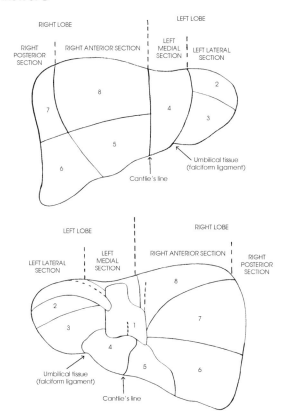

Question 36
Answer A

Question 37

Answer E – Other risk factors for HCC include cirrhosis, hepatitis B, alcohol, Wilson's disease, aspergillus and hepatocellular adenoma.

Question 38

Answer A – Arterial neoangiogenesis is the landmark pathological feature of HCC. Immunomarkers found in HCC are glypican 3 (GPC3), HSP 70 and glutamine synthetase (G3). Tumours can have a distinct fibrous capsule.

Question 39

Answer E – The bright dot sign refers to the presence of a bright dot within a lesion that remains hyperattenuating on arterial and portal venous phase CT. It is most commonly found in hepatic haemangiomas.

Question 40

Answer C

Non-cirrhotic patients with HCC – up to 50% liver resection is possible.
Medical – Sorafenib – not licensed by NICE
Symptom control – Furosemide + Spironolactone
Procedural –

TACE – Trans arterial chemoembolisation

- o Large doses of chemotherapy injected into arteries supplying tumour
- o Artery then embolised with foam or coils
- o Can be given multiple times
- o Contraindicated in renal failure + decompensated liver disease

SIRT – Selective internal radiotherapy

- o Form of brachytherapy
- o Glass beads coated in radioactive yttrium
- o Injected into tumour via hepatic artery
- o Use in palliation + bridge to surgery

Ablation – Radiofrequency ablation is standard method. Also ethanol, RAF + TACE for maximum benefit.

Irreversible electroporation (IRE) –

- o Uses nano-knife

o   When tumour near major vascular structures

o   Causes cellular apoptosis

Surgery

Liver resection – Only for non-cirrhotic or Childs A

Question 41

Answer B – All the other options represent relative contraindications rather than absolute.

Question 42

Answer E

Question 43

Answer C

Pre-sinusoidal	Sinusoidal	Post-sinusoidal
Portal vein thrombosis	CIRRHOSIS	Budd–Chiari Syndrome
Splenic vein thrombosis	Viral hepatitis	Veno occlusive disease
Schistosomiasis	Alcoholic liver disease	
Hyperdynamic splenic circulation (splenomegaly)	Primary biliary cirrhosis	
	Primary sclerosing cholangitis	
	Haemochromatosis	
	Wilson's	

Question 44

Answer B – The Child–Pugh classification incorporates bilirubin, albumin, prothrombin time, ascites and hepatic encephalopathy. The MELD (Model for End-stage Liver Disease) score is an algorithm using bilirubin, creatinine and INR.

Question 45

Answers:

1 – c

2 – d

3 – a
4 – f
5 – h
6 – i
7 – g
8 – e
9 – j

Interpretation of Hepatitis B Serology Test Results							
HBsAg	HBV DNA	HBcAb (IgM)	HBcAb (IgG)	HbeAg	HBeAb	HBsAb	Interpretation
–	–	–	–	–	–	–	Susceptible to HBV infection
✓	✓	✓	✓	✓	–	–	Acute HBV
✓	✓	–	✓	+/-	+/-	–	Chronic HBV (> 6 months)
–	–	–	✓	–	–	✓	Immune to HBV (past infection)
–	–	–	–	–	–	✓	Immune to HBV (vaccinated)

CHAPTER 14 – COLORECTAL SURGERY

Question 1

Answer C – Initial management of a shocked patient due to any cause is resuscitation. In this case, shock secondary to bleeding cross match is appropriate. Tranexamic acid is an antifibrinolytic agent which acts by binding with plasminogen. This prevents plasmin and preserves fibrin matrix. Intravenous administration of tranexamic acid is appropriate to control haemorrhage. Urgent CT angiogram with a view to consider angioembolisation is appropriate. Bowel preparation is contraindicated and colonoscopy in the initial stages is futile.

Question 2

Answer C – Anal ulceration needs urgent assessment by examination under anaesthetic to rule out anal cancer. The pathology may simply be primary fissure in ano. Lateral sphincterotomy in this case is not the initial management option. Topical medications to relax internal sphincter is most appropriate management. Stopping nicorandil is appropriate. Nicorandil is well known to cause anal ulceration. Manual anal dilatation should never be performed.

Question 3

Answer E – Acute poucitis is a common complication in pouch patients. Initial management is always conservative. Most of the cases respond to oral metronidazole and or ciprofloxacillin. Pouch excision is a last option, incidence of this is around 10% in the long term. VSL #3 has been shown to be beneficial in chronic pouchitis.

Question 4

Answer C – Anastomotic leak following low anterior resection varies between 5–15% dependent on the level of anastomosis. WCC and CRP levels are not reliable, can be normal even if there was anastomotic leak. Almost all patients with anastomotic leak will have associated ileus and atelectasis. It is important to rule out the leak and not to assume the pyrexia is due to atelectasis. Anastomotic leaks can be managed with laparoscopic approach provided there is expertise. Not all anastomotic leaks need complete dismantling of the anastomosis. In selected cases, anastomosis may be preserved with pelvic wash and a drain.

Question 5

Answer B – Best current treatment for anal cancers is combined radiotherapy and chemotherapy. Combined treatment has been proven to be superior to radiotherapy alone. Treatment failure is very small. Despite presence of inguinal lymph node, initial chemo-radiotherapy is the treatment of choice. Persisting anal caners are treated by salvage AP resection often with plastic surgical reconstruction including excision of posterior vaginal wall excision.

Question 6

Answer A – This vasculopathic patient is likely to have ischaemic colitis or even ischaemic bowel, either small bowel or large bowel due to raised WCC, acidosis and raised lactate. Following resuscitation, patient should have CT scan assessment to understand the site of vascular obstruction, to plan the surgical intervention. Interventional radiology is indicated where ischaemia is not suspected and to angio-embolise bleeding from the gut. Colonoscopy is contraindicated where gangrene of the colon is suspected. If adequate perfusion has been demonstrated on CT angiogram and the patient is haemodynamically stable, colonoscopy without any bowel preparation would help assess the severity of ischaemic mucosa. Use of therapeutic clexane is indicated where ischaemic colitis has been diagnosed and other conditions such as ischaemic small bowel and large bowel have been ruled out.

Question 7

Answer D – Patients with FAP should have colonoscopic screening early on, as early as 10 years of age. By 40 years most patients would have developed bowel cancer. Desmoid tumours are well known to be associated with FAP patients. Dependent on the location, abdominal desmoids may hinder the formation of ileal pouch. FAP patients are also prone to develop gastric and duodenal polyps, hence gastroscopic surveillance is also essential. Commonest cause of death in FAP patients is colorectal cancer followed by duodenal/periampullary cancer.

Question 8

Answer B – Recurrent rectal cancer is a rare, but challenging problem. PET scan is essential to rule out the metastatic disease prior to embarking on major surgical resection. S3 involvement and sacral foramen involvement is not a contraindication for excision.

Question 9

Answer D – GTN treatment for acute fissure in ano is initial treatment of choice. The results are approximately 60% healing at 6 weeks. Internal sphincterotomy has more than 90% cure rates. In the long term, patients treated with GTN have poor outcomes and compliance rates are approximately 50%. GTN acts by vasodiating by increasing the local concentrations of nitric oxide. This also relaxes the smooth muscles, thereby increasing the local oxygen for the fissure in ano for healing.

Question 10

Answer B – In multiparous women, risk of incontinence should be kept in mind; hence conservative management is the correct initial management of choice. In patients who fail conservative management and have low anal canal pressures, excision of the fissure with flap reconstruction is a recognised treatment option.

Question 11

Answer D – Elderly patients with incontinence are often managed conservatively. Initial assessment with history and examination is mandatory. Conservative management after flexible sigmoidoscopic assessment to rule out any left colonic pathology is appropriate. Sphincter repair is more successful in young women especially post-obstetric injuries, but futile in the elderly. Dynamic grac**i**loplasty is also reserved for the young and a select group of patients. Colostomy is last management option in this patient.

Question 12

Answer D – A very large proportion of colorectal cancers express cycloxygenase 2 (COX 2) than COX 1. Anti-inflammatory drugs such as aspirin and sulindac have been shown to reduce incidence of colorectal polyps and hence colorectal cancers. There is no evidence that ingestion of multivitamin pills reduces the incidence of colorectal cancers.

Question 13

Answer D – Patients suspected to have HNPCC should have genetic counselling. MSI tested from the tumour samples. CHRPE is not relevant in the HNPCC, but in FAP. Prognosis is better in HNPCC colon cancers than sporadic cancers.

Question 14

Answer A – Patients with first-degree relatives under 40 should be considered for baseline colonoscopy and referral to genetic counselling. There is no indication for regular aspirin intake. Reducing red meat and increasing fruits, vegetables and fibre intake has been shown to reduce colorectal cancers in the long term. There is no role of vitamin D in the prevention of colorectal cancer.

Question 15

Answer C – Ileo-anal pouch surgery can be performed in this patient after thorough counselling and education. It is essential to make sure that there is no Crohn's disease in the histology. There is definite reduction in fertility after pouch surgery. It is always advisable for patients to complete their family before considering pouch surgery.

Question 16

Answer B – Incidence of desmoid tumours is 10% in patients with FAP. Small-bowel polyps may be diagnosed by small-bowel enteroscopy. Retinal examination is useful to check for congenital hypertrophic retinal pigment epithelium. NSAIDs do not eradicate rectal cancer risk but have been shown to reduce it.

Question 17

Answer B – High ligation of IMA pedicle has not been shown to be beneficial and is thus not essential. Routine rectal wash with cytocidal solution has not been clinically proven to be useful; however, this is a standard practice. Anastomotic leaks are not prevented by defunctioning ileostomy. Surgeons should aim for 5cm of distal clearance below the tumour margin for a poorly differentiated tumours and 2cm for well differentiated tumours. For distal rectal cancers 1cm margin is considered adequate.

Question 18

Answer A – Gastrointestinal stromal tumours are rare tumours of the GIT. Most common site of the GIST is stomach. These are more common in patients with neurofibromatosis. Other sites are small bowel and rectum, which is believed to be more aggressive. Tumour size more than 5cm, high mitotic index, high cellularity predicts poor prognosis. Metastases are usually in the liver and lungs through haematogenour route. Tyrosine kinase inhibitors such as imatinib (Glivac) are very effective. Second line therapy includes sunitinib (Sutent®) and regorafenib (Stivarga). Medical therapy helps to reduce the extent of resection.

Question 19

Answer A – Follow-up after colorectal resections is not suitable for patients who have poor functional status. As per BSG guidelines (2002) follow up helps detection of early recurrences, the finding of metachronous disease (5–10%), facilitation of audit and the addressing of any surgical complications that happen early in the follow-up period. FACS randomised controlled trial concluded that the advantages are small with 3–5 years of follow-up with CEA and CT scans. Early diagnosis of local recurrence following rectal cancer resection is quite challenging, often requiring several investigations including biopsies and PET scans.

Question 20

Answer E – Colorectal cancer screening has been shown to be a very effective strategy to pick up early cancers and has been shown to reduce mortality. FIT test is superior to FOB, with higher sensitivity. For patients with HNPCC, colonoscopy is the best option as right-sided tumours are more common.

Question 21

Answer C – HNPCC is associated with colorectal cancers and extra colonic tumours. Autosomal dominant condition. HNPCC is of two types. Lynch syndrome type 1 (cancer site specific) and Lynch syndrome type 2 (cancer family syndrome) are the two types of HNPCC. The cancers occur at an early age, affecting predominantly the right colon. In type 2 Lynch syndrome, there is high risk of extra colonic cancers especially endometrial cancers (40%). Retinal pigment abnormalities are noted in patients with FAP but not in HNPCC.

Question 22

Answer E – Not all AIN III will progress to anal cancer. Natural history of anal intra-epithelial neoplasia is uncertain unlike cervical intra-epithelial neoplasia (CIN) where the risks of malignant transformation is over 30% from CIN III. The incidence of progression of AIN III to cancer is less predictable than that of CIN III. All types of AIN III are generally excised, as a standard treatment of choice. Radiotherapy or chemotherapy is not indicated. Routine histological assessment of haemorrhoidal tissue is not a standard practice; however, if AIN III is detected in the haemorrhoidal tissue, then follow up will simply be like other cases of AIN III with close surveillance to monitor. Anal cancers and AIN are associated with human papilloma virus (HPV) types 16, 18. Common skin warts are associated with HPV types 1 and 2.

Question 23

Answer D – Patients with long term constipation needs investigations such as MR defecating proctogram and NM colon transit studies to rule out slow transit and local pathology such as rectocele and rectal intussusception. Initial management after negative colonoscopy is to initiate treatment with diet and conventional laxatives. Patients with history consistent with IBS-C need to be on a LOW FODMAP diet. Often with this, many patients notice improvement in symptoms. If this fails, consider colonic prokinetic agents such as H5T-4 agonists such as prucalopride (Resolar). There are other medications such as linaclotine (Constella), a guanylate cyclase-C receptor agonist that increases bowel secretions and movement. Subtotal colectomy is never a choice for these patients.

Question 24

Answer C – Colonic ischaemia is a concern post-operatively in patients who had AAA repair. In most cases, the management is expectant unless the frank gangrene of the sigmoid has been proven on the investigations. Very unstable patient, with high lactate, WCC beyond 25 all point to significant ischaemia. In such cases, exploration may be necessary. Where patient is stable, flexible sigmoidoscopy is attempted to assess colon. Tranexamic acid is contraindicated in this scenario.

Question 25

Answer D – Septic picture following pouch anal anastomosis needs urgent investigations more commonly to rule out leak or pelvic collection, or even pouch ischaemia in rare cases. Usual modality of investigation is CT scan with pouch contrast to look for leak and collection. Pelvic collections need to be drained urgently. In the majority of cases, a temporary ileostomy would have been carried out; this is indicated where there was no prior diversion. Extremely rarely, a pouch excision for ischaemia may need to be carried out. Unfortunately, diverting ileostomies do not prevent a leak from the anastomosis. Early pouch-related sepsis predicts subsequent failure leading to pouch excision (1% per year).

Question 26

Answer E – Lymphomas are rare tumours of the gastrointestinal tract. 3% of all gastric tumours are lymphomas. Treatment of H. pylori is thought to cure some patients with gastric lymphomas. However, high-grade gastric lymphomas are treated by chemotherapy (CHOP regimen). Gastric perforation is a risk in such patients who are treated with chemotherapy. Small-bowel lymphomas are similarly rare after adenocarcinomas and neuro-endocrine tumours (NET). MEN-1 syndrome is associated with gastrinomas. T cell lymphomas of the small bowel are associated with malabsorption enteropathy such as coeliac disease.

Question 27

Answer C – Gastrointestinal stromal tumours are rare non-epithelial mesenchymal tumours. GISTs represent less than 1% of all GI tumours. Initial management is Glivec, to which approximately 80% of patients respond. Small-bowel and rectal GISTs are both more aggressive than gastric GISTs. Small-bowel GIST is generally treated by surgery.

Question 28

Answers:

A – 4
B – 3
C – 3
D – 10
E – 7
F – 8
G – 6
H – 1
I – 5
J – 10

Question 29

Answers:

A – 1
B – 3
C – 4
D – 5
E – 2

Question 30

Answers:

3 – A. Acute abdomen on day 5 following bowel resection is strong indicator of anastomotic leak. This should never be assumed to be due to ileus or chest infection, which is often the reason for delayed diagnosis with poor outcomes. Raised CRP of over 150 on day 5 with raised lactate is a strong pointer to anastomotic leak; these supplement clinical findings. Urgent investigations and abdominal exploration are indicated to save patient.

2 – B. Patients who undergo extended right hemicolectomy are more prone for ileus especially if gastric sleeve resection has been carried out. Other factors contribute to ileus including open surgery, prolonged surgery and the drugs tricyclic antidepressants, Lomotil, opiates, antihistamines.

1 – C. Atelectasis is one of the commonest post-operative complications. Clue in this case is early rise of temperature with tachypnoea without much abdominal signs.

5 – D. Generally patient after colonic anastomosis tachycardia on the 5th post-operative day should raise suspicion of leak. CRP of 200 on day 5 and raised WCC is a clue. Non-peritonitic abdomen is clue for small leak. However, urgent CT abdomen with rectal contrast is indicated. Careful monitoring versus surgical intervention options are weighed based on the patient's background and co-morbidities.

4 – E. Predisposing factors for pneumonia in this case are open surgery and poor pain control secondary to long incision. Associated COPD increases risk of pneumonia significantly.

Question 31

Answers:

A – 3
B – 4
C – 2
D – 1
E – 6
F – 5
G – 9
H – 10
I – 8
J – 7

CHAPTER 15 – VASCULAR SURGERY

Question 1

Answer B

Question 2

Answer A – ESVS guidelines recommend interval scanning every two years. All others should be considered for intervention.

Question 3

Answer C – As per NICE guidelines

Question 4

Answer E – This is a cross femoral venous bypass procedure that is often only utilised in threatened limb viability (phelgmasia).

Question 5

Answer E – In a salvageable but threatened limb, the most likely cause would be a brachial emboli, which would best managed with an embolectomy.

Question 6

Answer E – Avoiding a general anaesthetic would be favourable in this situation. Whilst heparin should be utilised, it is unlikely to result in restoration of inline flow. Catheter directed lysis can be performed under local anaesthetic and permits intervention on the likely underlying graft stenosis.

Question 7

Answer E – Whilst options 1, 2 and 3 are possible in this setting, the most likely cause for loss of arterial flow is popliteal occlusion due to intimal vessel damage and thrombus formation in the context of blunt force knee trauma.

Question 8

Answer C

Question 9

Answer C – Also known as "effort thrombosis", this is the consequence of venous thoracic outlet syndrome resulting in axillo-subclavian vein thrombosis.

Question 10

Answer A – Distal hypoperfusion ischaemic syndrome (a.k.a. steal) in relation to the creation of a proximal arteriovenous fistula

Question 11

Answer A – Stenoses of <50% or those with occlusion do not meet criteria for intervention. Stenoses of the CCA are not routine indications for surgery, even in the presence of symptoms. 'Younger' male patients with significant stenoses are considered to gain most benefit from CEA, as the stroke risk reduction occurs over the following five (plus) years. Therefore, if the patient is unlikely to survive this duration, any benefit will be lost.

Question 12

Answer A – Staphylococcus, frequently as part of a biofilm with or without resistance. Antibiotic treatment is often targeted towards gram-positive organisms as a consequence.

Question 13

Answer C – Frequently owing to plaque rupture

Question 14

Answer D – This is likely to be an infected aneurysmal transformation of fistula. Clinical situation above describes a 'herald bleed', which mandates urgent admission and intervention.

EXTENDED MATCHING

Question 15

Answers:
A – 1
B – 8
C – 6
D – 3
E – 10
F – 9

Question 16

Answers:
A – 6
B – 4
C – 1
D – 8
E – 2
F – 9

Question 17

Answers:
A – 1
B – 2
C – 4
D – 5
E – 3
F – 4

Question 18

Answers:

A – 3
B – 9
C – 4
D – 9
E – 7

Question 19

Answers:

A – 1
B – 3
C – 6
D – 7

Question 20

Answers:

1 – D
2 – E
3 – A
4 – B
5 – B

CHAPTER 16 – TRAUMA SURGERY

Question 1

Answer A – Activated protein C. Studies have shown that patients admitted in ATC have levels of aPC 5 times higher than in those with normal coagulation. High aPC is associated with increased fibrinolysis by consuming plasminogen activator inhibitor-1 releasing tPA from its inhibitory control. 'ROTEM' stands for rotational thromboelastometry and is used for diagnosing trauma induced coagulopathy.

Question 2

Answer C – Below the renal arteries at the point of the bifurcation of the aorta. B is Zone 2 and A is Zone 1.

Question 3

Answer D

Question 4

Answer D

AAST Renal Injury Scale		
Grade*	Injury type	Description of injury
I	Contusion	Microscopic or gross hematuria, urologic studies normal
	Hematoma	Subcapsular nonexpanding, without parenchymal laceration
II	Hematoma	Nonexpanding perirenal hematoma confined to renal retroperitoneum
	Laceration	<1 cm parenchymal depth of renal cortex, without urinary extravasation
III	Laceration	>1 cm parenchymal depth of renal cortex, without collecting system rupture or urinary extravasation
IV	Laceration	Parenchymal laceration extending through renal cortex, medulla and collecting system
	Vascular	Main renal artery or vein injury, with contained hemorrhage
		Segmental infarctions without associated lacerations
V	Laceration	Completely shattered kidney
	Vascular	Avulsion of renal hilum, which devascularizes kidney

*Advance one grade for bilateral injuries up to grade III

Question 5

Answer C – Renal trauma is treated much more conservatively than even 10 years ago. The key is to retain renal function as much as possible. Even with a renal artery embolisation, retroperitoneal collaterals should help to retain some function of the kidney.

Question 6

Answer D – And potentially try to realign facial anatomy with epistats, dental blocks and a hard collar.

Question 7

Answer E – This is an unsurvivable injury with likely diffuse axonal and brainstem injury. The poor prognostic features are bilateral blown pupils and no improvement with hypertonic saline.

Question 8

Answer C – The AIS is an anatomical-based system of coding developed by the Association for the Advancement of Automotive Medicine and represents the threat to life. It represents the type, location and severity of the injury. For more in-depth information see: https://www.aaam.org/abbreviated-injury-scale-ais/.

Question 9

Answer B

Question 10

Answer A

Question 11

Answer A

Question 12

Answer D – Tranexamic acid is an antifibrinolytic drug. An additional 1g IV bolus can be given in a situation such as the above scenario.

Question 13

Answer C – Anterior to the midaxillary line to avoid the long thoracic nerve of Bell and over the rib to avoid the neurovascular bundle that follows all the ribs. It is also important to administer a prophylactic dose of antibiotics.

Question 14 – Trauma Techniques

Answers:
1. C
2. B
3. A
4. E

5. F
6. H
7. J
8. D

The Kocher manoeuvre is used to mobilise the duodenum and access the head of the pancreas. Its use is limited in a trauma laparotomy but an isolated pancreatic head laceration from a penetrating injury may utilise this technique. It can be extended along the white line of Toldt and line of fusion of the small bowel mesentery to provide right medial visceral rotation and expose most of the retroperionteal structures of the abdomen. A Mattox manoeuvre is used for left medial visceral rotation and is especially useful when controlling the supracoeliac aorta to control a supramesocolic haematoma. A Pringle manoeuvre is used to clamp the portal vein, hepatic artery proper and CBD and can be used to gain control in severe hepatic haemorrhage.

A cardiac tamponade isn't suitable for pericardiocentesis as the clotted blood won't evacuate, so a left anterolateral thoracotomy should be sufficient. This can be extended into a clamshell thoracotomy if required, which should be used when managing injuries to the great vessels as greater visualisation is provided through the larger incision.

Pre-peritoneal packing is used to control bleeding from a pelvic fracture as the majority are venous in origin. Blunt lateral retroperitoneal haematomas should be managed conservatively.

Question 15 – Burns

Answers:
1. A
2. D
3. C
4. B
5. E
6. F
7. H
8. G

The Wallace Rule of Nines is a common, quick way to calculate the extent of burn injuries. It is more extensive than the Palmer technique of using the patient's hand, but less than the Lund and Browder chart. The Parkland formula is frequently used to calculate the required volume of fluid for resuscitation.

Superficial burns do not penetrate into the dermis. Partial thickness injuries affect the dermis to varying degrees; the more superficial ones tend to be excruciatingly painful and have small blisters associated with increased blood flow to the area. When the haemoglobin extravasates due to injury to the capillaries in the dermis, it gives the blotchy appearance seen in deep dermal injuries which often heal poorly. Full thickness burns eradicate the dermis and are insensate with a waxy or leathery appearance, commonly with eschar formation. The Jackson model describes the pathophysiology of a burn, whilst the Curreri formula calculates calorific requirements following burn injury.

Question 16 – Trauma Figures

Answers:
1. D
2. F
3. A
4. H
5. H
6. C
7. C
8. F
9. G
10. E

The cardiac index is a measure of the cardiac output from the left ventricle to the body surface area per minute. Several studies have been performed comparing the efficacy of external and internal chest compressions in animal and human models with variable results but internal cardiac massage produces a far greater cardiac output.

The AAST models for liver and spleen injury stratify the degree of injury by the proportion of subcapsular haematoma. Less than 10% is grade I; more than 50% is grade III.

Liver
Grade I

- o Haematoma: subcapsular, <10% surface area
- o Laceration: capsular tear, <1cm parenchymal depth

Grade II

- o Haematoma: subcapsular, 10–50% surface area
- o Haematoma: intraparenchymal <10cm diameter
- o Laceration: capsular tear 1–3cm parenchymal depth, <10cm length

Grade III

- o Haematoma: subcapsular, >50% surface area of ruptured subcapsular or parenchymal haematoma
- o Haematoma: intraparenchymal >10cm or expanding
- o Laceration: capsular tear >3cm parenchymal depth

Grade IV

- o Laceration: parenchymal disruption involving 25–75% hepatic lobe or involves 1–3 Couinaud segments

Grade V

- o Laceration: parenchymal disruption involving >75% of hepatic lobe or involves >3 Couinaud segments (within one lobe)
- o Vascular: juxtahepatic venous injuries (retrohepatic vena cava / central major hepatic veins)

Grade VI

- o Vascular: hepatic avulsion

Spleen
Grade I

- o Subcapsular haematoma <10% of surface area
- o Parenchymal laceration <1cm depth
- o Capsular tear

Grade II

- o Subcapsular haematoma 10–50% of surface area
- o Intraparenchymal haematoma <5cm
- o Parenchymal laceration 1–3cm in depth

Grade III

> o   Subcapsular haematoma >50% of surface area
>
> o   Ruptured subcapsular or intraparenchymal haematoma ≥5cm
>
> o   Parenchymal laceration >3cm in depth

Grade IV

> o   Any injury in the presence of a splenic vascular injury* or active bleeding confined within splenic capsule
>
> o   Parenchymal laceration involving segmental or hilar vessels producing >25% devascularisation

Grade V

> o   Shattered spleen
>
> o   Any injury in the presence of splenic vascular injury* with active bleeding extending beyond the spleen into the peritoneum

Injury Severity score ranges from 0 to 75 and uses the three most severely injured body regions to calculate the value. 16 and over is considered to be major trauma.

TABLE 2. Sample Injury Severity Score (ISS)

Body region	Injury	AIS*	Top three AIS scores squared
Head/Neck	No injury	0	
Face	No injury	0	
Thorax	Flail chest	4	16
Abdomen	No injury	0	
Extremity	Femur fracture	3	9
External	Contusion	1	1
Total ISS			**26**

* Abbreviated Injury Scale.

The Glasgow Coma Score measures the degree of unconsciousness from 3 to 15.

Glasgow Coma Scale		
Response	Scale	Score
Eye Opening Response	Eyes open spontaneously	4 Points
	Eyes open to verbal command, speech, or shout	3 Points
	Eyes open to pain (not applied to face)	2 Points
	No eye opening	1 Point
Verbal Response	Oriented	5 Points
	Confused conversation, but able to answer questions	4 Points
	Inappropriate responses, words discernible	3 Points
	Incomprehensible sounds or speech	2 Points
	No verbal response	1 Point
Motor Response	Obeys commands for movement	6 Points
	Purposeful movement to painful stimulus	5 Points
	Withdraws from pain	4 Points
	Abnormal (spastic) flexion, decorticate posture	3 Points
	Extensor (rigid) response, decerebrate posture	2 Points
	No motor response	1 Point
Minor Brain Injury = 13-15 points; **Moderate Brain Injury** = 9-12 points; **Severe Brain Injury** = 3-8 points		

50% of blunt trauma in the UK is due to falls, whilst 30% is due to motor vehicle collisions.

CHAPTER 17 – BARIATRIC SURGERY

Question 1
Answer D

Question 2
Answer A – Many bariatric surgeons would accept GORD and Barrett's oesophagus as a contraindication for sleeve gastrectomy with most considering Barrett's oesophagus as an absolute contraindication.

(Rosenthal, R.J., International sleeve gastrectomy expert panel consensus statement best practice guidelines based on experience of >12,000 cases. *Surg Obes* Relat Dis. 2012; 8(1): 8–19.)

Question 3

Answer D – Patients with an active psychiatric disease, a recent suicide attempt, personality disorders or drug/alcohol dependency are not suitable candidates for surgery until appropriately treated; these are considered as an absolute contraindication (while active disease).

It is important to assess individual patients in a multidisciplinary approach to ensure appropriate patient selection and assess risk–benefit profile in the individual patient. The other options in this question are relative contraindications and patients have to be assessed on an individual basis. For example, Crohn's disease itself is not an absolute contraindication to bariatric surgery, but would be a contraindication for a malabsorptive procedure. A sleeve gastrectomy is a preferred option for cases with Crohn's disease.

Question 4

Answer D – A history of smoking in a patient after a gastric bypass should alert to the presence of marginal ulceration at the GJ anastomosis. If the patient presents with signs of sepsis, the most likely diagnosis is a perforation of the GJ anastomosis. Other risk factors for marginal ulceration are the chronic use of NSAIDs, steroids and H. pylori infection.

Question 5

Answer A – A CT scan with oral contrast will help characterise the site of perforation.

Question 6

Answer D – An omental patch repair is the most common way of treating a perforated marginal ulcer after a gastric bypass in the acute setting. For chronic complications, such as strictures or intractable ulcers, a GJ resection and redo or even a gastric bypass reversal might be required.

Question 7

Answer E

Question 8
Answer C

Question 9
Answer A

Question 10
Answer A – There is a considerable amount of vitamin B12 stored in the body, so a deficiency takes more than a year to develop after the lack of absorption. With regards to folate, the risk of severe deficiency is quite low, because folate is produced endogenously within the body by the gut flora. Unlike the other deficiencies, thiamine deficiency may have an early onset after surgery if there is persistent vomiting and rapid weight loss, with a decrease in thiamine serum levels, since the half-life of thiamine reserves is from 9 to 18 days.

Question 11
Answer B

Question 12
Answer E

Question 13
Answer A

NICE guidelines for bariatric surgery:

1. BMI of 40 kg/m2 or more,

2. BMI of 35 kg/m2 or more with obesity-related co-morbidities e.g. diabetes, hypertension, sleep apnoea, PCOS

3. BMI of 30–34.9 who have recent-onset type 2 diabetes
   (In Asian population: the use of lower BMI threshold of 27.5 kg/m2 is considered for patients with recent onset type 2 diabetes)

AND all of the following:

- All appropriate non-surgical measures have been tried but the person has not achieved or maintained adequate, clinically beneficial weight loss.

-   The person has been receiving or will receive intensive management in a tier 3 service.

-   The person is generally fit for anaesthesia and surgery.

-   The person commits to the need for long-term follow-up.

Question 14
Answer D

Question 15
Answer C

Question 16
Answer D – When assessing a patient with an adjustable gastric band (AGB) with acute onset of symptoms, we have to exclude complications arising from the AGB such as a tight band, band slippage or erosion. A plain abdominal X-ray is useful to assess the position of the gastric band. A phi angle (angle between a vertical line orientated along the spine and one along the long axis of the gastric band) of more than 58° would indicate a slipped band. A vertical position of the band or a band oriented in a 4–11 o'clock position are also indicators of band slippage, as well as an 'O' sign [O-shaped configuration of the gastric band].

An endoscopy is usually useful to assess for gastric band erosion. The initial management would include accessing the subcutaneous band port to aspirate the fluid from the band. Surgery is usually the next step and options include removing the gastric band or adjusting the band position.

Question 17
Answers:
1) G
2) C
3) D
4) A
5) F
6) B
7) H
8) E

Question 18

Answers:

1) C
2) E
3) B
4) F
5) A
6) G
7) D

Question 19

Answers:

1) G
2) F
3) A
4) C
5) E
6) B
7) D

CHAPTER 18 – BREAST SURGERY

Question 1

Answer C – ASCO guidelines recommend HER2 targeted therapy for HER 2 positive disease with either sequential or concomitant chemotherapy.

Radiotherapy is indicated after breast conserving surgery and reduces locoregional recurrence and mortality. Contraindications include pregnancy, inability to tolerate positioning for treatment or previous radiotherapy to site.

Table 1: Breast Cancer T, N, and M Categories

Primary Tumor (T):

TX: Primary tumor cannot be assessed
T0: No evidence of primary tumor
Tis: Carcinoma in situ (DCIS, LCIS, or Paget's disease of the nipple with no tumor mass)
T1: Tumor is ≤2 cm
T2: Tumor is >2 cm but <5 cm
T3: Tumor is >5 cm
T4: Tumor of any size growing into the chest wall or skin

Lymph Node Status (N):

NX: Nearby lymph nodes cannot be assessed
N0: Cancer has not spread to nearby lymph nodes
N1: Cancer has spread to 1 to 3 axillary lymph nodes, and/or tiny amounts of cancer are found in internal mammary lymph nodes on sentinel lymph node biopsy
N2: Cancer has spread to 4 to 9 axillary lymph nodes under the arm, or cancer has enlarged the internal mammary lymph nodes
N3: One of the following applies:
- Cancer has spread to 10 or more axillary lymph nodes
- Cancer has spread to the lymph nodes under the clavicle
- Cancer has spread to the lymph nodes above the clavicle
- Cancer involves axillary lymph nodes and has enlarged the internal mammary lymph nodes
- Cancer involves 4 or more axillary lymph nodes, and tiny amounts of cancer are found in internal mammary lymph nodes on sentinel lymph node biopsy

Metastases (M):

MX: Presence of distant metastases cannot be assessed
M0: No distant spread
M1: Spread to distant organs is present

DCIS: ductal carcinoma in situ; LCIS: lobular carcinoma in situ.
Source: References 6, 12, 21.

Question 2

Answer B – Ultrasound is very reliable in the diagnosis of fibroadenoma in the under-25-year age group in which the incidence of breast malignancy is very low. A biopsy can be avoided if the ultrasound features indicate fibroadenoma. Patients can be reassured and discharged with advice to return if there is a change. Ten percent of fibroadenomas may increase in size following diagnosis.

Fibroadenomas are benign lesions that do not transform into malignancy. Simple fibroadenomas can be removed if symptomatic and patient wishes to undertake the procedure. Removal of fibroadenomas causing discomfort should be carefully discussed as the surgical wound can also cause discomfort post operatively.

Question 3

Answer A – After gliomas, meningiomas and schwannomas, pituitary adenomas are the most common benign intracranial brain tumour. Most of these are clinically non-functioning (i.e. non-hormone producing) or prolactin producing. Patients can present with gynaecomastia, galactorrhoea and visual field disturbance (bitemporal hemianopia) as a result of the presence of a prolactinoma. Treatment of the prolactinoma, either pharmacologically or surgically, should lead to resolution of gynaecomastia.

Question 4

Answer D – Tamoxifen is a selective oestrogen receptor modulator. When binding to oestrogen receptors in mammary tissue it has an inhibitory effect blocking the proliferation of oestrogen receptor positive breast cancers. Tamoxifen is the most common endocrine therapy agent in pre-menopausal women with hormone receptive tumours and is usually prescribed for a minimum of 5 years. It is not uncommon for women to experience changes in their menstrual cycle while taking tamoxifen including complete cessation while taking tamoxifen. This may be secondary to the medication itself but may also indicate menopause. Where the latter is suspected, FSH levels will be persistently raised.

Aromatase inhibitors have a limited role in oestrogen receptor blockade in breast cancers of pre-menopausal women. When ovarian secretion of oestrogen ceases, aromatisation of testosterone in peripheral tissues becomes the primary source of oestrogen which aromatase inhibitors can block.

Aromatase inhibitors have been used as a cross over medication where patients may have received 2 years of tamoxifen before menopause. The ATAC study and BIG – 198 study demonstrated the superiority of aromatase inhibitors over tamoxifen in increasing disease-free status in post-menopausal women. Local protocols dictate which aromatase inhibitor is used in postmenopausal patients.

Question 5

Answer B – Fibroepithelial lesions are usually cellular fibroadenomas or phyllodes tumours. Phyllodes tumours can be either benign or malignant. Differentiating one from the other requires histological assessment of the entire tumour into benign, borderline or malignant categories. Benign Phyllodes tumours require clear margins of >1mm. The evidence for the width of clear margins for borderline and malignant lesions is variable. Previous recommendations suggested 1cm but more recent evidence suggests clear margins are adequate regardless of width.

Question 6

Answer B – Literature suggests smear cytology sensitivities range from 11.1 to 16.7%, with specificities of 66.1 to 96.3%. This low PPV of smear cytology is partly due to a low epithelial cell yield at sampling.

Question 7

Answer C – The overall impact of adjuvant radiotherapy is a 50% reduction of any first recurrence. The absolute benefit is, however, less in older patients, with lower risk cancers.

Question 8

Answer E – Studies have also shown that at least one mutation is present in 59% of the Ashkenazi Jewish population. 4–5% of breast cancer is due to a predisposing gene. The LFSPD gene is associated with adrenal tumours. BRCA genes are associated with ovarian, prostate, pancreatic and colorectal cancers. Women with established breast cancer have a 2–5% risk of having cancer in the contralateral breast.

Question 9

Answer B – 18–20% of breast cancers overexpress the HER-2 receptor.

Question 10

Answer D – A sentinel lymph-node biopsy should be considered for patients undergoing mastectomy for DCIS, at the same time, as this technique cannot be used once the breast is removed. The node positivity rate in these patients is <1%.

Question 11

Answer A – The most important cancers detected at screening are high-grade DCIS, and grade 2 and 3 invasive breast cancers under 10mm. High-grade DCIS is likely to progress to grade 2 or 3 invasive breast cancer within the following 3 years. Grade 2 or 3 invasive cancers, when caught below 10mm, are much less likely to have metastasised.

Question 12

Answers:
1) E
2) D
3) I
4) A
5) G
6) G

CHAPTER 19 – ENDOCRINE SURGERY

Question 1

Answer B – Clinical presentation of PHP is very variable with the historic pneumonic – "renal (stones), abdominal (groans), psychiatric (moans)". Fatigue is the most common symptom present in >80%. Numerous studies have shown that a high percentage of patients originally thought to be asymptomatic actually do have occult symptoms upon direct questioning.

Question 2

Answer A – Single adenoma (up to 90%), multiple adenomas (up to 5%), hyperplasia (up to 9%) and carcinoma (<1%) can be considered as the causes for PHP.

Question 3

Answer B – With regard to pre-op localisation, the most sensitive is the sestamibi scan along with ultrasound of the neck, which would localise up to 80–100% with a specificity of 90%. MRI is best reserved for re-operation for localisation in PHP, where parathyroid scintigraphy is negative or equivocal.

Question 4

Answer D – This patient is presenting with hypercalcaemic crisis where aggressive IV fluids resuscitation should be the first step. This can be followed by loop diuretics, bisphosphanates (pamidronate more effective) and calcitonin depending upon serum calcium levels. Second-line therapy includes plicamycin, gallium nitrate, glucocorticoids and phosphates.

Question 5

Answer A – PHP is confirmed by elevated serum calcium and PTH levels. (iPTH) levels are highly accurate in diagnosing PHP. A chloride : phosphate ratio >33 is indicative of PHP in both hypercalcaemic and normocalcaemic patients. The presence of hypercalciuria rules out benign familial hypercalcaemic hypocalciuria, which can mimic PHP. Due to decreased resorption of phosphate by renal tubule, phosphate levels decrease in up to 50% of patients with PHP.

Question 6

Answer E – Other causes include tuberculosis, Paget's disease, milk-alkali syndrome, multiple endocrine neoplasia (MEN), familial hypocalciuric hypercalcaemia, and other medications such as thiazides.

Question 7

Answer C – The superior parathyroids are generally between the oesophagus and pharynx, while the inferior parathyroids are found in the anterior mediastinum and thymus. For ectopic glands, it is commonly the thymus. For missed glands, always check in the normal anatomic location.

Question 8

Answer D – When encountering an incidentaloma, the initial thing to establish is whether the mass is benign or malignant. Following this is the need to confirm if it is functional or non-functional.

Incidentalomas measuring more than 5cm need laparoscopic adrenalectomy irrespective of functional status as the chance of malignancy is high. CT-guided biopsy is only performed in case of history of previous malignancy to rule out metastasis. Once the mass is confirmed non-functional after routine biochemical work up, it can be observed with yearly scans to check for size increase.

Question 9

Answer D – Pre-operative workup for adrenalectomy should always start with alpha blockade followed by beta blockade. The patient is generally started a few weeks before the procedure with alpha blockers like phenoxybenzamine, followed by beta blockers like atenolol or propranolol. They should be extensively resuscitated with fluids pre-op, as post adrenalectomy can lead to sudden hypotension and hypoglycaemia.

Question 10

Answer B – Cushing syndrome causes elevation of almost all biochemical parameters except potassium, leading to hypokalaemia. It is described as hypercortisolism. It can be pituitary dependent arising from pituitary adenoma, which is more common than adrenal dependent resulting from adrenal adenoma. It can also be caused by ectopic ACTH-dependent secretion.

Question 11

Answer E – The commonest cause of Cushing syndrome is exogenous administration of steroids, which is most likely iatrogenic. Pituitary adenoma is the next common cause after iatrogenic administration followed by adrenal adenoma or bilateral hyperplasia. Ectopic secretion is rare.

Question 12

Answer A – The thyroid is supplied by the superior thyroid artery, which is a branch of the external carotid, and the inferior thyroid artery, which is a branch of the thyrocervical trunk, and sometimes by an anatomical variant, the thyroid ima artery.

Question 13

Answer C – Calcitonin is produced by the parafollicular cells of the thyroid gland. Serum calcitonin measurements are raised in case of medullary thyroid cancer. These are also used as tumour markers for the same. CEA levels are also used as a useful marker.

Question 14

Answer A – The radioactive scan characterises and determines the cause of hyperthyroidism. Even though US and FNAC of neck are critical, in cases of hyperthyroidism, the iodine uptake scan is primary as it helps distinguish between the causes.

Question 15

Answer E – Grave's disease is the commonest cause of hyperthyroidism. It is more common in women than men. It is an auto-immune disorder which involves TSH receptor antibodies along with thyroid peroxidase antibodies. ATDs such as carbimazole and methemazole are effective enough in achieving euthyroid state in most of the patients. β blockers are added along with potassium iodide (Lugol's solution) 10–14 days prior to surgery, which is also effective in a third of the patients. High-dose cholestyramine treatment up to 12 gms divided 3-times daily has also been reported. In case of thyroid storm, hydrocortisone at a dose of 100 mg every 8th hourly after a loading dose of 300 mgs, or dexamethasone at a dose of 2mg twice daily can be used.

Question 16

Answer D – Bethesda classification for FNAC results for thyroid ranged from THY1 to THY6:

THY1-non-diagnostic-rpt FNAC with U/S

THY2-benign-clinical follow up

THY3-atypia of undetermined significance or follicular lesion-Rpt FNAC

THY4-follicular neoplasm or suspicious of follicular neoplasm-Lobectomy

THY5-suspicious of malignancy-total thyroidectomy or lobectomy +/-frozen section

THY6-malignant-total thyroidectomy or lobectomy

Question 17

Answer E – Generally cold nodules are considered more suspicious for thyroid malignancy than hot. Young females with family history or h/o neck irradiation are considered high risk.

Question 18

Answer A – Papillary thyroid carcinomas account for 80% of thyroid cancers and carry a more favourable prognosis than other types. Follicular accounts for 15%. Both are considered as differentiated thyroid cancers. The remaining 5% are the undifferentiated or poorly differentiated thyroid cancers, which consist of medullary, anaplastic, lymphomas and metastatic lesions.

Question 19

Answer C – Patients <45 years old show excellent prognosis irrespective of nodal status and a small decrease in survival in the presence of metastasis. The highest stage for patients under 45 years of age is stage II. Staging systems include AMES (age, metastasis, extent, size), AGES and MACIS. The most commonly used currently is the sixth edition AJCC/IUCC staging system.

Question 20

Answer C – This patient has medullary thyroid cancer, which accounts for 5% of thyroid cancers and is hereditary or sporadic. It is now a disease characterised by RET proto-oncogene. Any patient diagnosed with MTC should be investigated for MEN 1 or 2 to screen for associated endocrinopathies like pheochromocytoma or hyperparathyroidism. Treatment for MTC is total thyroidectomy and bilateral central lymph node dissection (level VI). CEA is a useful marker along with calcitonin.

Question 21

Answer E – This patient is suffering from Hashimoto's thyroiditis (strong risk factor) for which she was on thyroxine replacement to encounter hypothyroidism. Now it has transformed into a lymphoma (non-Hodgkin B-cell type being the commonest), hence the night sweats, fevers and weight loss. For lymphomas, an open or core biopsy must be performed to establish diagnosis. The treatment for lymphomas is chemoradiation. The role of surgery is controversial and should be considered on an individual basis primarily for palliative debulking of compressive neck disease.

Question 22

Answer E – Insulinomas arise from the beta-cells of the pancreas. They are the commonest pNET (pancreatic neuro endocrine tumour) with least malignant potential (10%). Most insulinomas are single discrete tumours. A 72-hour fasting test is diagnostic to confirm insulinomas. In the setting of MEN1 (islet cell tumour of pancreas, pituitary adenoma or hyperplasia and parathyroid hyperplasia), they are more likely to have multiple tumours throughout the pancreas. Elevated serum calcium levels should raise the suspicion of MEN1 and parathyroid hyperplasia. Other pNET's like glucagoma and stomatostatinoma have the highest malignant potential (90%). Gastrinomas constitute around 70% and VIPomas 50%.

Question 23

Answer A – RLN injury should be <1% with accurate dissection. Up to 7% suffer transient vocal cord palsy secondary to surgical trauma and neuropraxia.

Question 24

Answer B – 131 iodine-metaiodobenzyl guanidine scan (MIBG) is the most commonly used for functional localisation to confirm diagnosis. Sestamabi scan is used for localisation of parathyroid adenomas. The specificity of CT and MRI for pheochromocytoma is limited. MRI is used more in children and pregnant women.

Question 25

Answer E – MEN I includes islet cell tumours of the pancreas (insulinomas, hyperparathyroidism and pituitary prolactinomas). MEN IIa includes medullary thyroid cancer, pheochromocytoma and hyperparathyroidism. MEN IIb includes medullary thyroid cancer, pheochromocytoma and mucosal neuromas.

Question 26

Answer E – The recurrent laryngeal nerve is most commonly posterior to the tuberculum. Options A, B and C are also possible locations.

Question 27

Answer D – The British Association of Endocrine and Thyroid Surgeons (BAETS) registry defines post-thyroidectomy hypocalcaemia as <2.1mmol/L on the first post- operative day.

Question 28

Answer A – Due to the high proportion of central lymph node involvement, a total thyroidectomy and central neck dissection is the mainstay of treatment.

Question 29

Answer E – Other suspicious radiographic findings are large tumours and irregular borders. The most common malignancy of the adrenal gland is metastases.

Question 30

Answer B – Between 75% and 80% of incidentalomas are non-functioning adenomas. The role of further investigations is to identify those tumours that are functioning or malignant.

Question 31

Answer D – They are described as Portland brick, which is a yellow/ brown colour.

Question 32

Answer A – Both the superior and inferior parathyroid glands have their blood supply from the inferior thyroid artery.

CHAPTER 20 – TRANSPLANT SURGERY

Question 1

Answers:

1. C. Banding – This is a working fistula with no evidence of tissue loss. Thus banding will be an appropriate first-line measure.
2. E. Radio-cephalic fistula. The minimum size to create a fistula should be at least 2.5mm and preferentially created on the non-dominant arm and distally.
3. K. Fistulogram. Prolonged bleeding is suggestive of venous outflow stenosis, which should be confirmed first by fistulogram to determine and plan treatment.
4. A. Ligate fistula – This is an actively bleeding fistula causing instability thus ligating would be the most appropriate. If the patient were stable, an interpostional graft could be considered.
5. H. Non-tunnelled lines. These are associated with the most infections and use should be minimised.

Question 2

Answer E – Brain stem death has to be confirmed by at least one consultant. No minimum time is set between the timings of the two sets of testing. It is not uncommon to have reflex spinal movements still present after brain stem death.

Question 3

Answer D – Treated cancer with no evidence of spread outside of the organ may be considered for transplantation.

Question 4

Answers:

1. D. Methylprednisolone. The first line of treatment for rejection is high dose steroids.
2. J. Retransplantation. Early hepatic artery thrombosis requires superurgent retransplantation due to the high rate of morbidity and mortality. There are case reports on attempts to revascularise the hepatic artery but currently this is done in only select cases.
3. G. Ultrasound. The first line investigation of transplant kidneys is ultrasound.
4. H. CT. Contrast CT to look for vascular compromise and evidence of pancreatitis.
5. Q. Nephrostomy. The priority here is to decompress the kidney and then investigate the cause of hydronephrosis.

Question 5

Answer C – The PD catheter should be removed as soon as possible together with the use of antifungal treatment.

Question 6

Answer B – Non-obese Type II diabetics may be considered for transplantation.

Question 7

Answer B

Question 8

Answer C

Question 9

Answer A – Up to 5 tumours under 3cm or a single tumour up to 5 to 7cm with no extra-hepatic spread are considered acceptable for listing.

Question 10

Answer D – Kidneys from donors who die from a stroke have a lower graft survival.

Question 11

Answer D – Selection for liver transplant is based on patients having a predicted 1 year liver disease mortality without a transplant of greater than 9% using the United Kingdom Model for End-Stage Liver Disease (UKMELD).

Question 12

Answer C – Though weight and gender mismatch between recipient and donor can result in poorer long-term outcomes, they are not currently used to allocate kidneys.

Question 13

Answer E – HLA matching is not routinely performed prior to liver transplantation.

Question 14

Answer D – Organ transplantation increases the risk of malignancy.

Question 15

Answer C – After reduction of immunosuppression, if the PTLD does not resolve rituximab may be used.

Question 16

Answer B – This patient requires their potassium correcting first through the placement of a temporary line to provide access for dialysis initially.

Question 17

Answer A – Tacrolimus levels go up with fluconazole, causing side effects such as tremor, headaches and graft dysfunction.

Question 18

Answer C – The treatment of BK virus is by the lowering of immunosuppression.

Question 19

Answers:

1) D. Veno-caval outflow stenosis causes ascites and oedema.
2) B. DCD kidneys are at higher risk of hepatic artery thrombosis.
3) A. Portal vein thrombosis occurs more in small children with hypoplastic veins.

CHAPTER 21 – UROLOGICAL CONDITIONS

Question 1

Answer A – In this age group, the likely diagnosis is patent processus vaginalis. Repair should be through the groin approach to identify and ligate the PPV sac. Repair through the scrotal approach will lead to a recurrence if the sac is not ligated. This can be confirmed with an USS prior to surgery, which will also identify a hernia.

Question 2

Answer D – This patient has a history of lower abdominal surgery and therefore closed SPC insertion is contraindicated. If no urology cover is on site he will need to be transferred somewhere with urology cover or have it performed under US guidance with an interventional radiologist. As he is in significant pain, the next step in your management would be to provide temporary relief by aspirating urine from the bladder with a needle up to 21G.

Harrison, S.C., Lawrence, W.T., Morley, R., Pearce, I., and Taylor, J. British Association of Urological Surgeons' suprapubic catheter practice guidelines. *BJU Int.* 2011 Jan.; 107(1): 77–85.

Question 3

Answer B – In the case of AUR, as the bladder expands it rises above the pubic symphysis. When safe to do so, in a distended bladder, in the absence of contraindications (mainly previous lower abdominal surgery or history of haematuria) an SPC can be inserted in the midline, using 2 fingerbreadths above the pubic symphysis as a landmark.

Question 4

Answer D – The layers of the testis are skin, dartos, external spermatic fascia, cremasteric fascia, internal spermatic fascia, tunica vaginalis, tunica albuginea which is adherent to the testis.

Question 5

Answer C – At around week 7 the medullary sex cord develops into sertoli cells which produce Mullerian inhibitory substance. This stimulates the first stage of testicular decent down to the level of the inguinal ligament and testosterone release from the Leydig cells. At around week 25, the second stage of descent is under the control of testosterone.

Question 6

Answer A – J. Oster demonstrated the natural history of the foreskin. At birth <5% foreskins retractile; ~5% non-retractile by 16 years.[1] This is in keeping with a physiological phimosis that traditionally appears as a 'pouting flower' on attempt to retract. BXO is very rare in children. Reassure the parents that the foreskin will eventually retract. An alternate option would be a trial of topical steroids. The indications for a circumcision include recurrent purulent infection of the prepuce, BXO, recurrent febrile UTI with abnormal urinary tract anatomy.[2] If there is evidence of redness to indicate a balanitis or balanoposthitis, this can be treated with a course of antibiotics.

1. J. Oster. Further fate of the foreskin. Incidence of preputial adhesions, phimosis, and smegma among Danish schoolboys. *Arch Dis Child*. 1968 Apr; 43(228): 200–203.

2. Statement from the British Association of Paediatric Urologists on behalf of the British Association of Paediatric Surgeons and the Association of Paediatric Anaesthetists. http://www.bapu.org.uk/wp-content/uploads/2013/03/circumcision2007.pdf.

Question 7

Answer C – This is an undescended testis as it retracts immediately on release. A retractile testis can be milked down to the scrotum and stays there – this can be managed conservatively. An ascending testis also requires an orchidopexy but is a phenomenon that occurs in children who previously had a descended testis. By 3 months of age, following a surge in luteinising hormone, testicular descent should have occurred. The operation can be performed between 6 and 12 months when the child is a little bigger and safe for a general anaesthetic. Once detected, a plan should be made for an orchidopexy and should not be delayed.

The BAPU Consensus Statement on the Management of Undescended Testes. http://www.bapu.org.uk/wp-content/uploads/2013/03/UDT-Summary-document.pdf

Question 8

Answer E – A, B and C would be associated with a history of pain. Idiopathic scrotal oedema typical presents in small children aged 4–6 and is typically a painless swelling. In the absence of a history of pain or trauma this is the most likely diagnosis. A differential diagnosis would include a hydrocele which can be evaluated with a scrotal USS.

Question 9

Answer B – Findings of a large scrotal haematoma raise suspicion of a testicular rupture. If USS is available this can be performed urgently to confirm this. However, to look for "significant injury to either the testicle or para-testicular structures and exploratory surgery is recommended to salvage the testicle and reduce postoperative complications".

Lucky, M., Brown, G., Dorkin, T., Pearcy, R., Shabbir, M., Shukla, C.J., Rees, R.W., Summerton, D.J., and Muneer, A.; BAUS Section of Andrology and Genitourethral Surgery (AGUS). British Association of Urological Surgeons (BAUS) consensus document for the management of male genital emergencies – testicular trauma. *BJU Int.* 2018 Jun; 121(6): 840–844.

Question 10

Answer D – The AAST classification of renal trauma is essential knowledge for any surgeon working in a trauma unit setting. This image shows contrast outside of the collecting system passing into the surround peri-nephric haematoma. This is a Grade 4 renal injury.

Question 11

Answer A – This image is a plain pelvic X-ray after a retrograde urethrogram. The bladder has been displaced cranially by the pelvic haematoma and there appears to be a large distance between the bladder neck and the bulbar urethra. This is suggestive of a significant urethral injury in association with a pelvic fracture. However, contrast is within the bladder. The cause for this is either the sphincter is now closed and no contrast is within the prostatic urethra or the contrast in the bladder has been excreted renally following the CT trauma scan that the patient will have inevitably had. In this case, it would be reasonable to gently try and pass a 12 fr urethral catheter under aseptic conditions. If there is any resistance or clinical concern then the next safest option would be to do an open cystotomy and supra-pubic catheter insertion at the time of his X-Fix.

Question 12

Answer E – The entire right kidney is devascularised. This is a Grade 5 renal injury suggestive of either a thrombosis or intimal flap of the main renal artery. If identified ASAP then an attempt at revascularisation may be considered by the vascular team/ interventional radiologist.

Question 13

Answer A – This lady has an infected and obstructed right kidney due to a large proximal ureteric stone. Her fever and AKI are concerning, in particular when considering her diabetes. She needs resuscitation, cultures, antibiotics and prompt surgical decompression. The literature suggests there is little difference in outcomes between a nephrostomy or a stent. In this case her being on apixiban is a contraindication to a nephrostomy and so a GA cystoscopy and right JJ stent insertion would be the most appropriate next step. Lithotripsy and primary ureteroscopy are contraindicated in infected systems.

Question 14

Answer D – The presence of bilateral renal stones in a child should always alert you to the likelihood of a metabolic cause. Her strong family history would make cysteinuria the most likely cause of her stones. This is caused by a defect in the COLA transport protein in the proximal renal tubule. It is inherited in an autosomal recessive fashion and causes high levels of cysteine in the urine, which is poorly soluble in urine.